How to
Prepare Now

Larry Deal

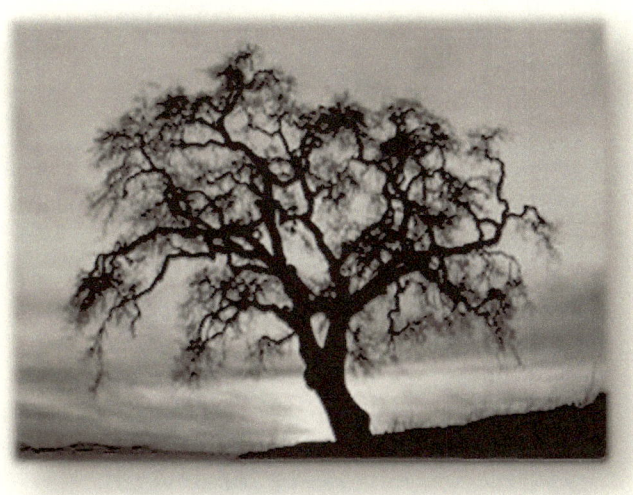

"If you cut down more trees than you grow, you run out of trees. If you put additional nitrogen into a water system, you change the type and quantity of life that water can support. If you thicken the earth's CO2 blanket, the earth gets warmer. If you do all these and many more things at once, you change the way the whole system of planet earth behaves, with social, economic and life support impacts. This is not philosophy, nor speculation, this is high school science. We've now passed the limits so we need to get ready for what's coming."

"In all this, there is a surprising case for optimism. As a species, we are good in a crisis and passing the limits will certainly be the biggest crisis our species has ever faced. Our backs will be up against the wall, and in that situation we have proven ourselves to be quite extraordinary. As the full scale of the imminent crisis hits us, our response will be proportionally dramatic. This is why I don't despair in the face of the science – it is precisely the severity of the problem that will allow us to realise our next great evolutionary potential, and that will drive a response that is overwhelming in scale and speed and will go right to the core of our societies."

From <u>The Great Disruption: Why the Climate Crisis will Bring On the End of Shopping and the Birth of a New World</u> by Paul Gilding.

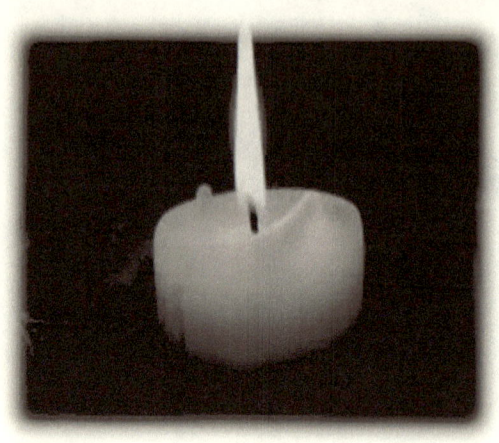

Disclaimer

I did a lot of research from many different sources for the material for this book. I apologize for not noting all these references. Many of the ideas came from the internet, from chat forums and blogs. These ideas came from real people with real experiences. A lot of the ideas came from my own intuition and experimentation. I encourage you to do your own research. Use this book as a catalyst to explore your ideas. I believe that every word in this book is true. My advice is to question everything you read that doesn't ring true for you.

CONTENTS

DEDICATION

This book is dedicated to my wonderful family, Carolyn, Grayson and Lacey who provide me with unconditional love on a daily basis. Their support is unwavering and gives me the motivation to think and create outside of the box.

ACKNOWLEDGMENTS

Thank you to my brother, Tony Deal, for his valuable help with this book.

Thank you to my sister-in-law, Jeany Bartlett, for her help with suggestions and guidance.

Thank you to my friend, Craig Miller, for spending his vacation time reviewing and making positive comments.

Thank you to my son, Grayson, for designing the cover and helping with the editing.

Thank you to Angela Lanyon for research and helpful suggestions.

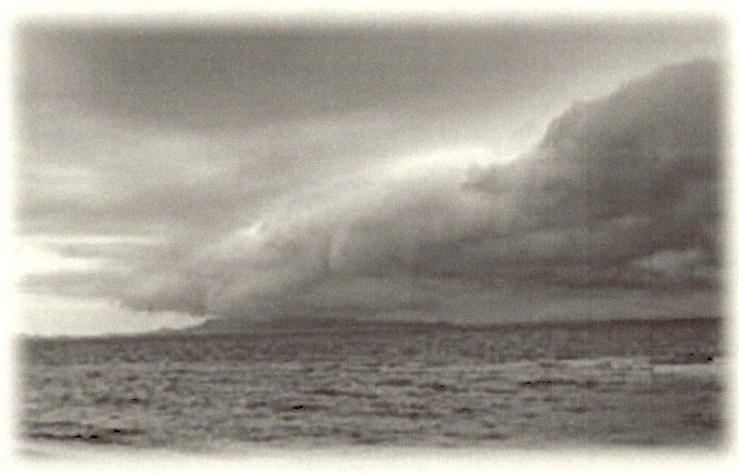

Chapter 1

Prepare *Now*

Preparing *now* for an anticipated disaster is the **smartest** thing you can do for you, your family and for your friends. I don't know how to make it any clearer. This strong and true statement deserves repeating many times. But I will state it just once again.

Preparing *now* for an anticipated disaster is the smartest thing you can do for you, your family and for your friends.

All of us want to be safe and secure, and we want the

same for our family and friends. We want to make smart decisions, especially those that affect the ones closest to us. Most all of us are smart, but we don't always make the smartest decisions.

Here is your chance to make the smartest decision of your life.

We hope that life will maintain as is, and we will not experience any type of disaster or major emergency in our lifetime. Regardless of what we want or expect, being prepared makes **good old fashioned common sense**, no matter what the future brings. Using our common sense and intuition, we know that the odds are stacked against us. Our generation has been extremely lucky in avoiding any type of major disaster. No generation in the history of the world has escaped one. We might be the lucky generation, but we might not.

This is not about extreme choices. This is about common sense choices. You won't have to live in a cave or dig an underground bunker. If you prepare smartly, you can live comfortably in any kind of disaster that we may face. Should a major disaster occur, many will be more comfortable than others. Many will survive based on basic necessities. Many will not survive.

We have taken for granted our abounding resources. We

have forgotten that those resources keep us alive, and without them, we cannot live. I hope through reading this book, you will begin to appreciate what you have, and make a conscious effort to protect everything that is precious on this earth. It is my hope that you start examining what is truly important to you, and make preparations to protect it.

After considering the food choices in this plan, you may decide to incorporate them in your daily life *now*. These choices will enhance your life, bring you back in touch with your food, make you feel better about yourself and make you healthier.

This book provides you with the knowledge to make smart, informed choices. It is up to you to take it and run with it. When you consciously prepare, you enhance your life in the present, giving you peace of mind. This is the peace of mind that, in the event of any type of emergency, you will be prepared to survive comfortably and help save your loved ones in the process.

This book is about hope. It is about joy and health. It is about living in the *now* and fully experiencing every second we have on this earth.

My Epiphany

Three years ago, I was nervously sitting in a gas line in Black Mountain, North Carolina, waiting patiently and hoping. Hoping there was enough gas left in the tanks, by the time I got to the pump, to fill up my car. My son, Grayson, was in his car behind me, and my wife, Carolyn, was in her car behind him. I was watching as people were standing outside their cars, visibly agitated. This was August of 2008, and we had not been able to purchase gas the previous two days. Carolyn couldn't go to work the day before because of lack of gas. Grayson and I needed the gas to get to a contracting job we were doing. People were stranded on Interstate 40 trying to get home from vacations.

At this moment, I felt so helpless. I was at the mercy of an outside force that controlled my life. If I wanted to go somewhere, I had to have the gas to move me and my vehicle to my destination. Like everyone else, I was addicted to the gas pump. It controlled my life and everyone else's life around me.

It was then, sitting in my car alone, that I had this frightening thought.

"What if it were food?"

It sent a chill down my spine. What if I were waiting in line for food? How helpless would I be feeling if I were waiting in a

6

line, hoping to get the necessary food to keep my wife, my children, and me alive?   That chill running down my spine soon turned into a knot in my gut. I allowed myself a few moments to explore this sad and sickening feeling, just to let it sink in.

That is when I realized I had to prepare and gain control over my food existence. I knew I had little, if any, control over my ability to get gasoline or control my mobile existence. I bought a car, a Prius that gets 45-50 miles per gallon. I could lessen the impact a little, but I really had no control over it.

I could gain total control over my food existence just being smart, informed and by taking action. I began by studying, researching, and planning.   This is where the material for this book came.   That is where the "Prepare *Now*" plan was born.   I realized that the most efficient and economical way to prepare for the future is to start *now* with a few lifestyle changes. I realized I could easily make a plan to store some food. I also understood that storing food for an emergency was only the beginning. Being totally out of touch with my food source, I made a commitment to get in touch with my food and help others in the process.

Where does our food come from?

Our food is largely dependent on outside sources.   Much of our produce comes from California, Florida, Mexico and other foreign countries. It is even coming from China. Can you believe that several of the natural food grocery store chains sell "organic" food from China?

How much common sense does that make?

The lettuce on your salad is traveling 3,000 miles to your grocery store. The vegetables on your plate come from a communistic country over 7,000 miles away.

How the heck did this happen?

Are we so dependent on other people's decisions that we allow them to use our precious resources, gas and oil, to bring us food from so far away?

Doesn't that affect not only our food existence but our mobile existence as well?

Doesn't that make the price of gas and oil more expensive?

We know that oil is a commodity dependent on supply and demand. Simple economics says that if you spend large amounts of oil doing unnecessary things, you are causing more demand for the oil. This makes the oil price go up, which in turn makes our gas prices go up. Using our precious oil in this manner makes us more dependent on its existence.

Our food supply is related to oil in other ways. It takes a

huge amount of oil to produce the chemical fertilizers that farmers use to grow the same crop over and over again on the same piece of land. We know that we don't have to do that by simple crop rotation. But, that doesn't make short term economic sense to the large corporate farms that control our food. They refuse to let the land lay fallow, or out of production for the correct amount of time, allowing the soil to regain its life giving nutrients with another crop in its place. It is cheaper and more profitable to make the same land produce more food each year using chemicals.

Oil is also used to produce the pesticides and herbicides that farmers use to control weeds and bugs. Of course these same chemicals are destroying our bodies, our land and our water.

How the heck did this happen?

Were we asleep at the wheel?

You bet we were and most of us still are.

Have you ever heard of so many food allergies that we have today? People are allergic to peanuts, to wheat, to soybeans, to almost every type of food that is in existence. Where did that come from?

I am only 56 years old, but this is all new to me. I don't remember any of that when I was a child. I don't remember people dying because they ingested a food that contained a peanut, unless they actually choked on it.

Where did all these allergies come from? Many informed sources say they are the result of the large amount of chemical fertilizers, chemical pesticides, chemical herbicides and chemical hormones that we ingest daily with our food. These chemical toxins put our immune systems on high alert and cause reactions, which turn our immune system against our own bodies.

Where did all the cancers and other deadly diseases come from? Is that also related to our food? The Hunzakuts, a group of people in the Himalayan Mountains of Pakistan never get cancer. They are among the healthiest and longest living people in the world.

What is their secret?

The answer depends on whom you ask. Ask the scientists who are paid by the big pesticide companies, and they will say that these people are blessed with good genes. Or, they will say that they live in a less stressful environment.

Probably not the best answer. Those factors certainly play a part, but they do not explain the whole picture. More likely the answer is they grow their own organic food without toxic producing chemicals. And, they are in touch with their food, breathe clean air and allow nature to be their doctor.

That doesn't set well with big business. Many large corporations see that as an affront to their bottom line. When anything becomes profitable, it becomes subject to greed.

Good natural health is not profitable, but...

Health is in your control.

You are probably wondering what this has to do with preparing for the future.

If we are dependent on oil to grow our food, transport our food and preserve our food, our food existence is just as out of control as our mobile existence. And when something is out of our control, we are setting ourselves up for a disaster.

If the trucks don't run, our food will run out in one week.

Here is another statement that deserves to be repeated.

If the trucks don't run, our grocery stores will be completely out of food in one week.

Any multitude of reasons could cause the trucks to stop running... an oil shortage, terrorist attack, natural disaster, solar flares, pandemic or whatever. Most people in the United States will be out of food in just one week.

Think about that for a moment. That means that nearly 300 million people will not have access to the things that keep them alive.

What will happen then? I don't know and I don't even want to think about it. It troubles me to think about people in this great country reduced to standing in line for food handouts just to feed themselves and their family.

If you would like to know what might happen if the trucks stop running, read "One Second After" by William Forstchen. It is a well researched novel. It may be fiction, but it is based on the fact that an electromagnetic pulse, (EMP) could stop our trucks in their tracks. This is not just science fiction. An EMP is highly plausible, can be caused by solar flares, or could be manmade. EMP's are being researched to stop run-away vehicles and as weapons in our defense system. They exist and could be used against us or could be a part of a natural disaster. Forstchen's book is a good read and a wake-up call for some.

We are being boiled alive while blissfully enjoying the hot tub.

You know the story. If you drop a frog in boiling water, he will immediately leap out. But if you put the frog in lukewarm water and gradually increase the temperature to boiling, he will die without knowing what hit him. That is where we are right *now*.

It is time to get out of the hot tub and start taking control of your life.

Why not make a few small changes in your current lifestyle that will enhance your life *now*? These changes will make you healthier *now* and help you prepare for an uncertain future.

You have the power of *now*.

Many of you may have read <u>The Power of Now</u> or <u>A New Earth, Awakening To Your Life's Purpose</u> by Eckhart Tolle. If not you should. It doesn't tell you a thing about disaster preparation, but it emphasizes the fact that *now* is what matters. *Now* is the best time you will ever have in your life to do the things that you enjoy. *Now* is the time to do what you love. *Now* is the time to prepare for the future so you can keep enjoying a healthy and joyful lifestyle that everyone on this beautiful earth deserves.

<u>How to *Prepare Now*</u> encompasses many things that will enhance your life, *NOW*.

For example, when you follow the *Prepare Now* plan you will start making your own bread. You will learn to make, easily and effortlessly, whole grain breads with no artificial preservatives or ingredients. This will make you a celebrity among your own group of family and friends. Everyone loves good fresh bread, but very few people make their own. And you probably thought it was too hard to make. It's not, and you can make it *now*, enjoying the fruits of your labor, while training yourself to be less dependent on the outside world for your food.

Whole grains are the most economical and safest foods to store for future use. Whole grains can be stored almost indefinitely if you store them correctly. I remember reading that when the tombs of ancient pyramids were opened, grain was found to be buried with the king. Researchers were able to successfully germinate the grain seeds, which were 3000 years old.

Bread has been a staple for almost all of human existence. I'm sure you've heard the phrase, "Man can't live by bread alone." There is profound truth to that. But man can survive on bread alone for a period of time.

You won't have to count on bread alone. Bread will enhance your health and your lives, while you add other healthy foods to it. This book teaches you "common sense health values". These values are the core foundation to preparation.

Good food, good water and a good community make for a healthier you, whether you are preparing for a future emergency or whether you just want to take control of your life *now*.

Building a strong barter profile is an excellent example of how you prepare *now* for the future while enhancing your life in the present. In a real disaster, one that may last for months, bartering is your best friend. You can't or should not expect to provide everything for yourself. In chapter ten you learn how best to acquire the tools and skills to have strong bartering power. You will be ready with the tools and knowledge when the time comes, because you will already be doing it and enjoying the new lifestyle.

You will be preserving your own food. There is no cheaper way or safer way to store food for the future than dehydrating and canning food. The chapter on preserving your food takes you through the steps to start your own food preserving process *now*.

There is a chapter on growing your own food and doing it *now*. No matter where you live, house or apartment, you can start growing your own healthy food, indoors and out, year round. Nothing gets you more in touch with your food than growing your own. Nothing can give you more satisfaction or make you healthier than growing your own food. You will learn to grow your own food easily and effortlessly without fail. You can't grow all your food, but you can easily grow lettuce indoors for a healthy salad every day. There are simple easy to follow directions that will give you an instant green thumb. Your friends and family will be in awe at your success. Organic, healthy food will adorn your table.

Should there be any other kind?

By buying and reading this book, you are already on your journey.

Today you are starting a new and wonderful journey to a new way of life. Today is the first day of your new life. Make today count. Take the reins and take control over your food. You will be taking control over your health and bringing more joy to your life *now*.

Enjoy the trip and be healthy and happy!

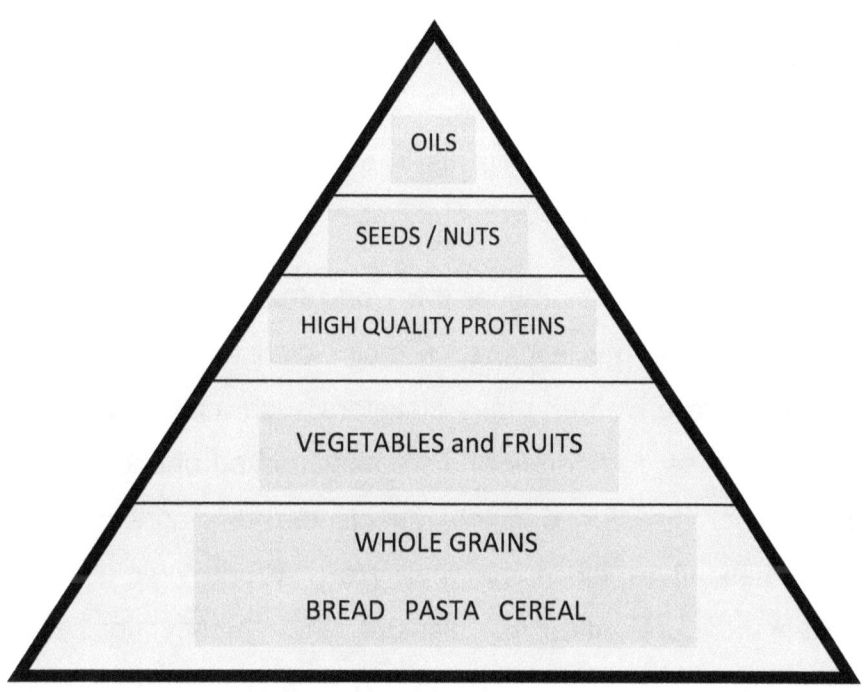

OILS

SEEDS / NUTS

HIGH QUALITY PROTEINS

VEGETABLES and FRUITS

WHOLE GRAINS

BREAD PASTA CEREAL

CHAPTER 2

Nutritional Food Plan

You must have some intuition that there could come a time when we will have to depend on our own resources to survive, or you would not be reading this book.   There seems to be that collective intuition among a lot of people, because I hear it almost daily. A recent poll depicted 41% of Americans believe that some sort of disaster is approaching. This collective intuition is the strongest reason I am preparing.

We are animals, and animals have the innate ability to predict a future disruption. Some think we have lost this ability. I disagree. There are many who hear the still small voice that attempts to communicate with us in a positive and protective manner.

Disasters have hit all over the world for many years, but the United States has escaped a major disaster in over 100 years. Yes, we have had many disasters such as Katrina and other hurricanes, tornadoes and weather related phenomena. But no major disaster, one that affects the very core of our society, has hit us since the Civil War. World War II was definitely a core affecting disaster, but mostly for the Europeans and Asians. The Civil War was the last major disaster on U.S. soil.

Are we due? Maybe. No one knows, but it will be very reassuring to be prepared just in case. The Great Depression in the 1930's was hard on America; however, America was more independent then. I asked my dad how he and his family fared in that depression, and this was his response.

"We didn't even know it was going on. We were already poor and had to rely on our garden and animals to feed us. Nothing really changed for us. We still ate the same food and life went on as usual".

This scenario would be very different if it happened now.

I am suggesting a new lifestyle change that may seem a little intimidating at first. But like any journey, it begins with a single step. Change is difficult for everyone, yet it is inevitable. Moving from a high stress, out of control existence to a simple lifestyle with less stress is positive change, which is much easier to accomplish. Change doesn't have to happen overnight, but if you start today and make a little progress each day, you will be way ahead of the rest. Gaining control over your life is a new beginning. Start today in a small way, because something could happen tomorrow. If you don't believe that, just ask the Japanese.

You could spend a lot of money buying prepared emergency food kits, but it is not necessary. Your grocery store is the place to start, and you can do it today.

This book is designed to help you provide healthy stored food at the lowest possible cost. Whole grains, dried beans, dried milk and cheese, dried whole wheat pastas, canned meats, canned vegetables, dried vegetables and dried fruits complete the food list.

A high level of nutrition for an emergency food storage system is essential. Many people will get more healthy nutrition from this emergency plan than their present diet. These small incremental lifestyle changes that can be built into your life today will prepare you for the future. When you start this plan *now*, you will move closer to your ideal weight and your ideal health.

You will feel better, have more energy and more confidence.

You body needs certain daily requirements from caloric intake. Protein, fiber, vitamins and minerals are all important to help keep us strong and healthy.

Phyto-nutrients, nutrients that build the immune system and protect against certain diseases are important in a daily diet. Food can be your medicine and your preventative medicine. In an emergency, a strong immune system is vitally important. Hospitals may be over run, doctors too busy to meet the demands put upon them, and the healthy will be needed to help others.

Now is the time to prepare your body for immune strength. Proper nutrition, proper exercise and the avoidance of the many health robbing foods which many of us indulge, such as highly processed sugars and flours, is essential. It is in your best interest to choose organic foods as often as possible. Pesticides, herbicides, genetically modified foods, hormones, antibiotics and steroids have all become part of our food system, causing a multitude of ills in our bodies.

Here is a brief description of each food category in the *Prepare Now* plan.

20

Dried Beans

Throughout history beans have been used as a staple of mankind's diet, and the health benefits derived from them have been well documented. They are full of nutrients, and the amount of nutrients per calorie is particularly high. Even though beans vary in color, size, flavor and shape, their nutritional content is very similar. One half cup of cooked dry beans contains approximately 115 calories and provides 8 grams of protein. Beans contain several types of phytochemicals, are rich in lignans, and have a low glycemic index. The properties of the carbohydrates found in dry beans, along with their fiber content, make them ideal foods for the management of abnormalities associated with insulin resistance and diabetes. They are also good for weight management.

Due to certain sugars contained in the beans, many people experience gas after consuming the beans. This can be greatly diminished by presoaking the beans overnight, discarding the water and cooking with fresh water. Black beans have much less of these gas-producing sugars than beans such as pintos.

Dried beans are rich in both soluble and insoluble fibers, helping to prevent constipation, colon cancer and other conditions that affect the digestive tract. They are very low in fat and very high in protein, containing 21-25% protein by weight. This is especially good for vegetarians who need more protein in their diet.

As for vitamins and minerals, beans are an excellent source of copper, phosphorus, manganese, magnesium and iron. They also provide the water-soluble vitamins thiamin and folic acid and are good source of riboflavin and vitamin B6.

Beans are included as an important part of the emergency food plan because they are very rich in nutrients, easy to store, high in protein, rich in fiber and are cheap. They are almost the perfect food, and when combined with whole grains, they become the perfect food.

Whole Grains

Whole grains have been an important part of our diet since early man. It is amazing that we have allowed ourselves to be duped into thinking that processed grains, which have the nutrients and fiber removed, as in white flour, is better for us. Many of us know that, but go into any grocery store and you will see 80% more white bread on the shelves than whole wheat. Go into a convenience store, and you usually can't find any whole grain bread. It is no wonder that our society is overwhelmed with problems such as obesity, cancers, diabetes and many other diseases.

Do you know how they process white four? Here's a quick lesson.

A wheat grain is composed of three layers...the bran, the germ and the endosperm. The bran is the outside layer where most of the fiber exists. The germ layer houses most of the nutrients, and the endosperm is the starchy middle layer.

Natural nutrition exists when all three layers are eaten together. Mills that grind whole wheat, grind it slowly resulting in flour with all three layers mixed in, thus whole wheat flour.

Enter white flour into the picture. Mass production uses high speed mills which remove the bran and the germ with the resulting flour being the starchy endosperm layer. The waste product, the bran and the germ, which of course is the most nutritious part, is sold as animal feed.

If that is not bad enough, the flour is then subjected to a chlorine gas bath. You may recall in your history class that chlorine gas was used in World War 1 to kill many people. Saddam Hussein also used chlorine gas to kill his own people in Iraq. Chlorine gas is a poison. Even the EPA identifies it as a powerful irritant, dangerous to inhale and lethal. The goal of using this gas is to bleach the flour, giving it the white pretty look.

Now they have nice pretty white flour devoid of any natural vitamins. Then they add back synthetic vitamin and mineral supplements to enrich it. Of course these synthetic vitamins are made from petroleum. Do you see an oil theme here?

OK. I will get off my soap box now, but I hope you can see why I have whole grains on the list. They are nutritious and healthy in their freshly ground whole natural state. And, they are much healthier for you when fresh ground. Flour loses a large percent of its nutrients two days after it is ground.

Whole wheat is not only delicious when baked into fresh bread,

It's good for you too.

Eating whole grains benefits your body in many ways. Studies show that whole grains can reduce risks of heart disease, stroke, cancer, diabetes and obesity

Whole wheat contains lots of fiber. Fiber can be thought of like a sponge for your body, scrubbing and cleaning the inside of the digestive system. It also makes you feel full, helping to regulate overeating. Whole wheat contains carbohydrates that provide energy and has an adequate amount of protein and antioxidants.

If you are allergic to wheat, there are other whole grains that have no gluten and are very good for you. Rice flour makes excellent bread, and there is always cornbread. You can research other grains and seeds that have no gluten that work just as well as wheat.

Oatmeal has strong health benefits. It is also inexpensive and stores very well, sealed with a vacuum sealer. There are many nutritional advantages of oatmeal. It is an incredibly rich source of dietary fiber. Along with fiber, it contains significant amounts of proteins, carbohydrates, vitamins and minerals. These vitamins and minerals include vitamin E, magnesium, manganese, copper, iron, selenium, calcium and zinc.

Oatmeal has many properties that may deter cancer, especially colon cancer. It lowers the bad cholesterol, thereby gaining its reputation as a **heart healthy food**. Oatmeal is also a good source of food for diabetics.

Whole corn has been a staple of the Native American diet for thousands of years. Columbus first discovered the use of corn by Native Americans and brought it back to Europe. It is a good source of many nutrients including thiamin (vitamin B1) pantothenic acid (vitamin B5), folate, dietary fiber, vitamin C, phosphorus, manganese and dietary fiber. It has been noted as a contributor to heart heath, not just for its fiber content, but for significant amounts of folate. You may recognize folate in ad campaigns to prevent birth defects. This B vitamin is important to our health in many ways. It has been estimated that consumption of 100% of the daily recommended requirement of folate could reduce heart problems by 10%.

Corn is a good source of protein and valuable calories in an emergency environment. It has been linked to increased memory function, prevention of colon cancer and reduced rates of lung cancer. It may even assist in preventing Alzheimer's disease.

Corn can be prepared in a variety of ways. With the addition of lime (calcium carbonate), as in the making of hominy, it can be even more nutritious. Making cornbread is easy and adds significantly to the enjoyment of dried beans. Add a little milk to cornbread and honey, and you have a great dessert.

You should purchase organic corn due to the high levels of pesticides and herbicides used to produce it and the fact that the majority of corn today is genetically modified. The only way that you can be assured of getting corn that is not genetically modified is to buy certified organic, unless you know the grower.

Flax Seeds

"Wherever flax seed becomes a regular food among the people, there will be better health."

... Mahatma Ghandi

Flax, although not technically a grain, has many of the characteristics of whole grains. However, its health-giving properties far outpace whole grains. Flax seeds complement grains for overall good health.

Early settlers knew the value of flax. It was grown for the high- quality cloth, linen, that the stalks could produce. It also produced linseed oil that was used for a variety of purposes, including a natural wood preservative. Flax seeds are low in carbohydrates, high in fiber, antioxidants and omega-3 fatty acids. Omega-3 fatty acids reduce inflammation in our bodies. There is plenty of research showing that inflammation plays a big part in diseases such as heart disease, arthritis, asthma, diabetes and some cancers.

Flax seeds help stabilize blood sugar and the high fiber content protects the intestines. They are high in phytochemicals, the disease fighting antioxidants. Flax is a great source of lignans, which help balance female hormones. There is mounting evidence that flax seeds can prevent breast cancer and type two diabetes.

Flax seeds must be ground in order for the body to assimilate it. They have a tendency to go rancid if stored in ground form, but the whole seeds store very well. You can easily grind them in a coffee grinder.

Eat Your Veggies

Fruits and vegetables lower the risk of heart disease, cancers, prevent digestive problems and contribute to overall good health. The dark leafy vegetables and colorful fruits contain the most nutrients. The best ways to consume vegetables and fruits are raw, lightly steamed, or quickly cooked in a pressure cooker. A great way to prepare vegetables for an emergency is to dry them for soups and add to grain dishes. Dried fruits can be eaten raw as a snack. The natural sugars are concentrated so they taste like candy. Dried fruits or fresh fruits, with a little addition of honey, make a great complement to oatmeal in the mornings.

You can grow vegetables year round. Spinach, lettuce and kale will grow any time of the year outside in most places in the United States, even in the cold and snow. When the weather gets extremely cold, a little plastic or glass cover will help them continue to grow and provide valuable food.

There is no reason to wait until a disaster to start your own small salad garden. You will immediately benefit from this valuable addition to your diet. It is not difficult and will help you get in touch with your food.

Nuts and Seeds

Raw nuts and seeds are a great enhancement to overall health. They are easily stored in the shell and can provide high amounts of protein and other nutrients. Seeds are not only good for you, but they are the life givers of next year's crop.

Seeds, under the right conditions, can survive for hundreds of years and still germinate to produce more seeds. There is evidence of seeds, thousands of years old, still having the ability to germinate. Most seeds will save in conditions around 70 degrees and 70% humidity or less for five years, so saving them is a great way to prepare for any disaster. Heirloom seeds are strongly recommended. You will be able to collect these valuable seeds every year.

Seeds can be sprouted for an explosive supply of nutrients. Some people believe that sprouts are the new fountain of youth. Sprouts are loaded with antioxidants, protein, vitamins, minerals and amino acids. Broccoli sprouts have been found to contain over 50 times as much of the antioxidant sulforophane than regular broccoli. Research shows that peanut sprouts reduce the bad type of cholesterol, and sunflower and grain sprouts aid people with diabetes.

Sprouts have the highest nutritional content of any food.

Sprouting is easy and important for an extra kick in nutrition. The easiest way is to buy a sprouting kit, but you can also use a jar, tray, or cloth bag.

You can sprout any seed, and every seed has its own distinct flavor. We have included three types of sprouts in this plan for the sake of simplicity and economics. These are clover, mung and chia.

Clover Sprouts

Clover is very similar to alfalfa sprouts, but with a sharper flavor. Clover sprouts are rich in phytochemicals. They contain genisten, which blocks the formations of blood vessels in tumors, essentially starving the tumor. These sprouts contain 26 % protein with the vitamins A, B, C, E and K. They are rich calcium, magnesium, potassium, iron, phosphorus and zinc. They contain naturally occurring estrogens, making them helpful with PMS and menopause.

Mung Bean Sprouts

Mung bean sprouts add a nice crunchy texture and flavor to salads. Among the cheapest high power nutritional foods you can buy, one pound of mung beans will develop 10 pounds of sprouts. As in all sprouts, mung beans are a nutritional treasure trove, aiding in disease prevention, building the immune system and relieving fatigue.

Chia Sprouts

Most people are familiar with chia as the novelty chia pet, being unaware that these seeds contain powerful nutrients. Known by the Indians of Mexico as the running food, chia was used as a high endurance food by the South and Western Indians.   Aztec warriors used it during long marches and in battle. It is a high source of protein and a muscle and tissue builder. One of the most profound properties of chia is its ability to absorb water, helping to prolong hydration.   There are so many advantages to consuming chia and chia sprouts that it could fill another book. Research this valuable seed on the internet, and you will grasp its amazing properties.

Peanuts

Peanuts, actually a legume, are an excellent source of protein, niacin and folate. They are high in energy calories, which is a good thing when storing food for an emergency. Peanuts store well and peanut butter has been known to be safe to eat after 25 years in a jar. Peanuts contribute to brain health, brain circulation and blood flow. High in antioxidants, peanuts protect against colon cancer, prostate cancer, breast cancer, heart disease and high cholesterol.

Meats

Meat is one of nature's most balanced foods. Loaded with necessary proteins and nutrients that keep our muscles and bones strong, meat gives us energy to do what we need to do to get through the day. Unless you are a strict vegetarian, meat will be an important part of your diet in an emergency. If you are a strict vegetarian, then you must work hard to find the right combinations of foods that give you the same necessary nutrients of meat.

Meats also store well. Dehydrated meat kept many explorers alive in our nation's early years. Jerky is simple to make, easy to store and packed full of valuable calories and nutrients. Canned meats, bought at the grocery, will store for many years. The process of commercial canning assures that the meat is properly processed so that botulism and other forms of bacteria are virtually eliminated. The shelf life of canned meat is long, some stating that 10 years is a good number, but I have heard of people eating canned meat over 60 years old. Many survival experts say that the contents will outlast the can, in other words the can will rust before the contents go bad. One thing is for sure, if the can is bulging, you would not want to eat the contents, an evidence of bacteria growing.

Canned fish, especially salmon, is an excellent nutritional choice for emergency food. Salmon has the essential oils and nutrients that improve our bones and organs, while enhancing our immune system. Be careful with tuna. Albacore tuna has too much mercury in it for good long term health. Regular dark tuna has much less and can be consumed in limited amounts without worrying about the negative effects of mercury on the body.

Sweeteners

Honey

Considered the perfect sweetener, honey is definitely the perfect storage food. It will keep for centuries and be safe to eat in just a jar with a lid stored in a cupboard. It contains vitamins and minerals, unlike zero-nutrient sweeteners, such as refined sugar. Honey is easily digested and contains antioxidants. Some people use it as a wound dressing to prevent bacteria growth. That alone is enough to include it in your emergency kit, but its greatest function is to increase quality of life. Emergency food doesn't have to be bland and boring. Honey can be added to oatmeal for a delicious breakfast and will be an important part of desserts.

Another essential sweetener is xylitol. This sweetener doesn't get the respect it deserves. Not only is this natural sweetener good for you, it protects your teeth against tooth decay. If you are not using toothpaste with xylitol, you should consider it *now*. Again, don't take my word for it. Do your own research. My research makes me a believer. The owner of a health food store tells me that people who use it bring her surprising stories about its value. There is no better resource than the testimony of real people.

Sugar is on the list mainly because it is cheap. Brown sugar is better, but white sugar is so cheap that you should store it, even if you use it for nothing more than barter.

Oils

Fats are an essential part of our bodies, and we must include them in our diets.   For the longest time, fats were considered bad for us, causing all sorts of problems from weight gain to heart disease. Now we know that fats are good for us, we just have to eat the right ones.

Too much fat in our diets does cause problems, but you won't have to worry about that in an emergency situation. French fries require too much energy and resources to make, putting them way down on the list of emergency foods. In an emergency, your oils will be precious, only to be used in salads and stir-frying foods.

The best oils for our bodies are olive oil, grape seed oil, safflower oil and peanut oil. Peanut oil is more stable at high heat, so it is the best oil to cook with. You can cook with grape seed, olive and safflower oil, but it's best to cook with them at lower heat settings.

Most oil crops such as safflower or canola are grown on huge farms with lots of herbicides and pesticides. It is best to buy organic if you can afford it. To make matters worse, these crops are mostly genetically modified. This allows for more pesticide and herbicides to be used. Genetically modified plants were modified to take more pesticides and herbicides without being damaged. They were also modified so that they would produce no viable seeds, so that the company that holds the patents on them (whoever thought we would allow a patent on a living organism) are the only ones with the reproducible seeds. This forces the farmers to buy new seeds every year.

These genetically modified plants are taking over the regular normal plants. They already account for over 95% of the corn produced and over 80% of soybeans and canola. They contaminate other heirloom and organic crops by cross pollination. Not only are the crops we feed our animals genetically modified, but the food we eat is also genetically modified. The huge agri-business companies have successfully lobbied to keep GMO identifying labels off our food. In other words, they prefer that we be ignorant about what we put in our bodies. As these plants take over our normal seeds, one of the traits that they contribute is the inability of the plant to reproduce. This so- called "suicide" gene trait may be good for the large agricultural companies, but could be devastating to the world. This grand experiment has humanity hanging in the balance. All our food sources could be in the control of a few large companies. If that doesn't scare you, I don't know what will.

How the heck did we let that happen? This is another reason to store seeds.

Oils should be stored in a cool dark place, such as your basement. Many oils go rancid in storage. Olive oil is your best storage oil, containing natural antioxidants that slow spoiling. Most other oils will go rancid in less than six months, even if kept correctly. Olive oil, stored in the basement can last two years. All oils should be kept in dark glass containers. If they are in clear bottles, wrap them with a cloth or put them in a covered box to keep out light.

When oils go rancid, they contain free radicals that can damage our bodies. For this reason, you should rotate your oils. Oils that you purchase in the grocery store should last for a year without going rancid. They have been treated with a preservative. You still want to make sure that they are stored properly.

Your Own Foods

This book is only a guideline to help facilitate your own personal nutrition preparedness program. Do your research into foods that you like and see if they make sense to add to your own plan. The internet is there for easy and effortless research into anything you want to know. I hope this book will be the catalyst to jump-start you on your own path to nutrition and preparedness.

There has never been so much free information on every subject imaginable as *now*. The internet is there for everyone, and you should use it to help formulate your plan of action. A word of warning though; it may not be there when you need it most. Create a file of all your information on your computer. Copy and paste, and file it on your computer so that it will be there when you need it. Make hard copies and keep them in a binder for easy reference. Reference materials will be great resources in an emergency. Books will be valuable to help keep you occupied and free from boredom

Want to lose weight? Most of us know that fad diets don't work. For a diet to be successful for the long-term, it can't be something you do; it has to be something you become.   .

Use the nutritional information and the menu section of Chapter 3 and form your own diet. Eat oatmeal every day with walnuts, fresh apples, flax seeds, honey and cinnamon. Have a 500 calorie lunch sandwich with whole grain bread and a nutrition packed middle loaded with fresh sprouts. Enjoy the great taste of fresh cooked dried beans and cornbread for dinner with a healthy salad.

When you give your body what it needs, cravings go away.   When the occasional craving does come, drink a glass of water, eat an organic apple and go for a short walk. As you walk and enjoy the beauty of nature, stand up tall with good posture and feel your body getting back to its normal healthy state. State a few positive affirmations about your new lifestyle.

Your body will thank you and reward you with health. Your brain will sense this healthy lifestyle and reward you with good feeling endorphins.

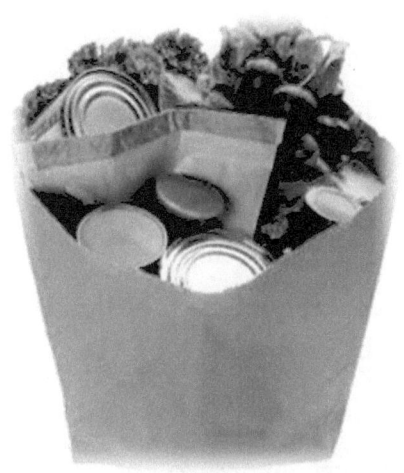

CHAPTER 3

What to Buy *Now*.

E veryone should start *now* collecting at least a three months food supply regardless of income. This book is for everyone. Some can afford to buy everything this book suggests. Some can only get the basics *now* and will have to accumulate the other things later.

Everyone can start *now* regardless of income.

If you are a single parent on food stamps, you can still prepare. Your selection may be limited, but you can store the correct foods that will provide the proper nutrition for you and your family to be healthy during a crisis. You will be doing what our ancestors have done for thousands of years… eating basic foods that are cheap and full of nutrition; beans, whole grains and meat.

The food groups important to your health are whole grain carbohydrates, proteins, vegetables and fats. You will get your vitamins and minerals from these groups. The great news is that they are available at your grocery store, packaged for long-term storage and ready to put in your kit. The other items that are essential for storage include things that will make your life more comfortable and food more enjoyable such as spices for cooking and personal items like toilet paper. You can buy everything you need to supply two people for three months for under $400. It is more economical to supply two people than for one person, because there is waste when you cook for just one person. More than likely, you won't be able to count on your refrigerator to store leftovers. This is a good reason to partner with others in your food storage program. If you live alone, *now* is the time to look into this situation and adjust accordingly.

A grocery list is at the end of this chapter. Your local grocery store can provide everything you need. Be sure to check local discount grocery stores for bargains. In Asheville, NC where I live, there are a few outlet stores that have amazing deals. One sells discount organic foods. These are perfectly good products with dented cans or ones bought at close-out sales. I can purchase whole grain rice meals there for fifty cents. I have seen these same meals in other grocery stores for two dollars. Check around and you will find lots of bargains.

Many of the foods on this list are prepackaged and ready for long term storage. Many are not. Items such as flour should be repackaged by you. You can take a five lb. bag of flour and put it in a vacuum seal bag to seal it from bugs, moisture and oxygen. These are the main causes of food deterioration. Keep in mind that bug larvae is probably in the flour when you buy it. Freeze it for a few days and add a little diatomaceous earth which will take care of the bugs. Adding an oxygen absorber will get rid of most of the oxygen that causes spoilage. A vacuum sealer will take care of that too. The O2 absorbers can be bought on the internet and are cheap, about ten cents each for a 100 cc packet. Read the instructions and you will know which size and amount you should use.

Let's get started. This is the basic list for anyone regardless of income or resources. Use this list as a guideline and add your own personal preferences.

Grocery List

Canned Meat

Meat provides protein, fats and a certain amount of vitamins and minerals. Canned meat can last for decades. There are reports of canned meat from the 1940's, provided in war rations for soldiers during WW II, that are still edible and in good shape.

If you like fish, you are in luck. Canned fish is packed with protein and contains the right amount of good fats for your health. And best of all, it is inexpensive. At my local grocery store, a twelve oz can of tuna packed in water cost only $2.49 and has sixty five grams of protein. That comes to only twenty cents an ounce. I have found five ounce cans of tuna for fifty cents a can. That's even cheaper. Salmon is a better bargain. A sixteen ounce can contains 105 grams of protein and only costs $2.00; 12.5 cents per ounce.

Chicken is a little more expensive, but still very reasonable. Ten ounces of canned chicken costs $2.00 and has forty eight grams of protein. Dried beef is more expensive at $3.39 for 4.5 ounces, with thirty two grams of protein.

You will be combining this meat with other less expensive foods, so the overall cost will be much lower than if you just use meat as your only protein source.

Dried Beans

Beans have been a staple of our ancestors for ions and for good reason. As I mentioned earlier in chapter two, dried beans are full of fiber and protein, store practically forever and are cheap. In an emergency situation, you will be eating them nearly every day, so get a variety. Lentils and split peas are quick and easy to fix. Black beans cause very little gas. Pintos are flavorful and cheap, and limas are full of vitamins and minerals.

Grains

You won't be buying whole grains for bread in the grocery store, but you can purchase whole grains in the form of pastas and cereals. I certainly recommend whole grains whenever possible, but there are exceptions to every rule. If you are getting plenty of fiber from other sources such as flax seeds and oatmeal, there is nothing wrong with eating macaroni and cheese. Mac and cheese is box-ready for long term storage, and most people, especially kids, like it. You should treat it like flour, and prepare it to protect it from pests and moisture.

Unbleached white flour is on the list for the purpose of making bread. It is not the ideal choice but keeps longer than whole grain flour. By all means, you should replace this with whole grain that you grind fresh everyday if possible.

Parboiled rice is on the menu. Brown rice doesn't store well and white rice is stripped of nutrients. Parboiled rice retains 80% of its nutrients and fiber, cooks quicker and stores well. Parboiled brown rice comes packaged as instant brown rice. Read the label to make sure it is brown rice. It is not really instant, requiring several minutes to cook. You can grind parboiled brown rice and add it to your flour for bread making.

Peanut Butter

There is probably no food that is cheaper, comes ready to store for years, and is packed with as many calories and protein as peanut butter.

Oils

I have included only olive oil in this list because of its ability to store well. You can add safflower, peanut oil or canola oil, just make sure you rotate them every six months or so.

Other Items

Jelly and preserves are on the list. Peanut butter and jelly sandwiches make an easy and calorie packed meal. I have included spices and staples that store well and will enhance any meal.

The $400 Plan

This plan is basic, but will provide good nutrition for two people for three months. It is a great place to start. Other things can be added later, but this week start buying enough food for three months. Spend a few dollars extra each week until the list is complete.

The menus may seem bland, and they are as compared to the meals you have access to today. In a disaster, good nutritional food will be valuable, even if it is repetitious and bland.

Bread is designed to go with these menus, but bread will not last for an extended period of time. Whole wheat flour will lose nutritional content and go rancid after a few months. White unbleached flour will last a few years, which is why it is included in the list. Freeze the flour for twenty four hours to kill any bugs that might be in it. Then repackage it in an airtight container with a few tablespoons of diatomaceous earth mixed in. Add a bay leaf. This will take care of the eggs and any small creatures that want to invade your flour.

Grains and a grain grinder are the only things necessary to add for maximum nutrition. Grains are not expensive, and you can pick up a hand grinder for under $50. To go with these, add forty pounds of bread grain, mainly wheat unless you are allergic to gluten. If so, research and you will find plenty of suitable substitutes. Corn is necessary for cornbread. Add forty pounds of dried whole corn. The internet and local mills are the best places to find them.

Always try to buy organic grains, but any grain is better than none. I can purchase a fifty pound sack of non organic dried corn locally for $8.00. It is genetically modified, and I personally don't care to put that stuff in my body. However, if that is all you can afford, then by all means, buy it and store it. It will keep you alive.

Dried corn has to be the cheapest food product you can buy. It only takes two cups or 3/4 of a pound to make a pan of cornbread. For $8 worth of corn, you can make sixty six pans of cornbread costing twelve cents for each pan. There are other ingredients, but even with those, a pan of cornbread will cost less than thirty cents. Below is a home ground cornbread recipe. It will be lighter and taste better if you substitute 1/2 cup whole wheat or unbleached white flour for 1/2 cup of the corn flour.

Great Tasting Cornbread Recipe

2 cups corn meal

1 tsp baking soda

1/2 cup wheat flour

1 1/4 cup milk (buttermilk is better)

1 egg

1 tablespoon oil

Mix all ingredients

Preheat oven to 450 degrees

Bake in a greased iron skillet for 15 –20 minutes

Serve with pinto beans and chow-chow for a healthy and delicious meal. For dessert, put a little honey over a piece of corn bread. I'll take that meal over anything our fast food restaurants have to offer any day.

Your Grocery List.

Remember this is a 90 day supply of food for two people. Add the correct amount for more people. This grocery list is based on a bare bones budget and something you can get started on *now*. There are a few important items I could not find in the local grocery store such as powdered eggs. You will find them on the internet.

This is also a guide. Use your imagination and your personal preferences. You will come up with what works best for you and your family. Just keep in mind the things that keep you healthy. Wherever possible, I chose items that come in glass jars instead of plastic. Some things such as ketchup are hard to find in glass. I also avoided food additives that are not healthy for you such as MSG and high fructose corn syrup. When I could, I avoided GMO products, which is nearly impossible. If you find a product that advertises non GMO products, you should buy that, even if it is more expensive. Baking powder is one of the items that advertised as a non GMO product and was aluminum free. Aluminum should be avoided whenever possible. That is why I do not cook in aluminum cookware.

A one a day multivitamin is also recommended. Natural and organic with whole food supplements are best. Choose the one best for your age group and gender.

Grocery List

Item	Price	Size	Amount	Total
Pintos	2.14	32oz	1	2.14
Split Peas	0.76	16oz	2	1.52
Small Red Beans	1.4	16oz	2	2.80
Black Eyed Peas	1.28	16oz	2	2.56
White Navy Beans	1.18	16oz	2	2.36
Lentils	0.94	16oz	2	1.88
Black Beans	1.96	32oz	1	1.96
Instant Brown Rice	1.26	14oz	10	12.6
Macaroni and Cheese	0.64		16	10.24
Spaghetti Pasta	2.72	48oz	2	5.44
Spaghetti Sauce	1.33	26oz	12	15.96
Canned Tuna	0.64	5 oz	24	15.36
Canned Salmon	2.48	14 0z	12	29.76

Canned Chicken	1.98	12.5oz	28	55.44
Sugar	3.08	5lb	1	3.08
Olive oil EVOO	18.64	101oz	1	18.64
Powdered Milk	18.28	4lbs	2	36.56
Mayonnaise	2.68	32oz	1	2.68
Dried Parmesan Cheese	2.62	8oz	1	2.62
Ketchup	1.78	35oz	1	1.78
Egg Noodles	1.5	12oz	2	3.00
Pickle Relish	1.68	16oz	2	3.36
Bread Crumbs	1.08	15oz	4	4.32
Chicken Stock	1.78	32oz	12	21.36
Vinegar	2.84	1 gal	1	2.84
Corn Meal Mix	2.28	5 lbs	2	4.56
Oat Meal	2.48	42oz	6	14.88
Peanut butter	3.67	26.5oz	3	11.01
Jelly	2.58	32oz	2	5.16
Macaroni and Cheese	0.36	Box	22	7.92
Unbleached White Flour	3.47	5lbs	6	20.82

Salt	0.34	26oz	10	3.40
Pepper	0.60	4	2	3.00
Garlic Powder	0.74	2.4oz	4	2.96
Mustard	1.26	24oz	1	1.26
Cocoa	2.42	8	2	4.84
Salsa	1.98	24oz	4	7.92
Baking Soda	0.52	1lb	2	1.04
Baking Powder	1.82	8oz	2	3.64
Yeast	4.14	4oz	2	8.28
Multi Vitamin	7.68	200	1	7.68
Bleach	2.98	1.4gal	2	5.96
Toilet Paper	6.47	24 rolls	1	6.47
				$388.94

Menus

Breakfast

Oatmeal cost $2.48 for a forty two oz. box which gives you thirty (150) calorie servings. For a 300 calorie breakfast, we will add a few things to the oatmeal. Sugar, milk and oil add calories and taste as well. Sugar is something to avoid in our modern world today, but in a disaster it can be invaluable. It is also cheap.

Oatmeal makes a great inexpensive nutritious breakfast, but most people will not eat it plain. Add a tablespoon of sugar to it and it becomes much more palatable. Honey is much better and more nutritious, but that is relevant to your budget. Regular white sugar is the cheapest sweetener. Powdered milk adds to the taste and adds valuable calcium and other nutritious calories. Add three tablespoons of powdered milk to each serving. Olive oil adds calories and valuable oil that your body needs. In a disaster we won't be counting calories to reduce them; we will be more concerned about counting them to increase them. If you have some dried fruit or walnuts, you can really increase the nutritional value and taste. Again, this is a budget issue.

Recipe

½ cup oatmeal cooked according to directions on box (150 calories) cost $.09

If you don't have the directions, just add water and cook it a few minutes, five minutes is usually enough.

At the end of cooking, add 3 tablespoons powdered milk, mixed with equal amounts of water. (50 calories) cost $.19

Add 1 tablespoon sugar (45 calories) $.02

Add 1 teaspoon olive oil   (40 calories) $.01

Salt to taste

Total calories   295 calories

Total Cost for Breakfast is $ .31

3 Month supply of breakfast for two people... $20

Breakfast is simple and cheap.   You can eat the same thing every day and not get tired of it. It is fuel for the first part of the day. Be creative and add valuable nutrition and healthy foods to start your day.   Adding dried fruit and nuts, which store very well, make a great addition to oatmeal. Flax seeds would be one of the most important things to add to oatmeal. I do it every day *now*. Be sure to grind your flaxseeds so that your body can utilize it well. A cheap coffee grinder will suffice.

If you or someone in your family doesn't like oatmeal, then be creative. Cold grain cereals store pretty well. Any whole grain cereals provide a good nutritious breakfast.

Ground flaxseeds, dried fruit and nuts will make cold cereals even better nutritionally. Of course you will need more dried milk and will have to adjust accordingly.

Lunch

Lunch is another simple meal. Our lunch goal is to provide nutritious fuel for our bodies in the easiest and cheapest form. Again it will be repetitious, but it will be invaluable in an emergency for your family. We are striving to get a certain number of nutritious calories into your body so you can function during the day without getting weak. We are targeting 500 calories for lunch. Some people will require more, some less. It depends on what your activity will be during the rest of the day. If you are working hard, then of course you will need more calories. If you are just resting and passing the time, you will need less. Men typically need more, women less.

I am assuming that you will be making your own bread as

laid out in chapter five. This is essential, because it makes lunch simple and easy. Sandwiches for lunch are nutritious and inexpensive. Our homemade bread accounts for approximately 140 calories per slice, so one sandwich already has 280 calories before you add anything to it. A tablespoon of peanut butter adds eighty calories and a table spoon of jelly adds another fifty calories. That peanut butter and jelly sandwich becomes nearly a full meal at 410 calories. When you add macaroni and cheese as a side, you get another 150 calories for a total of 560 calories for lunch. The cheap box-type macaroni and cheese will require some of your powered milk and olive oil to make it taste better. You will have this lunch four days a week.

Chicken salad or tuna salad will be on course for the other three days. If you are raising chickens or can barter for some eggs, this will be more nutritious and will taste better. If not, you can buy powered eggs, or make it with just mayonnaise and pickle relish. Tuna salad with just mayonnaise (one tablespoon with two 5 oz cans of tuna and pickle relish) is about 115 calories per serving and combined with the bread totals 395 calories. Add a side of parboiled rice (forty calories) with three tablespoons of powdered milk (fifty calories) and one teaspoon of olive oil (forty calories) and you just added 130 calories to the lunch. This nutritious lunch contains 525 calories. Chicken salad adds twenty more calories, because chicken has more fat than tuna.

If someone in your family doesn't like tuna or chicken salad, they can have another peanut butter and jelly sandwich. Get creative with their food tastes and create a special menu for them.

Lunch costs considerably more than breakfast, but you are getting more calories and more protein. Protein is more expensive than carbohydrates.

Dinner

For dinner, you can be more creative. I am still adhering to a cost efficient approach, but dinner is a time for relaxing and enjoying a good meal. One thing that will be on the menu every day is beans. Beans are the most cost effective food you can buy and provide many of the nutrients that you need. You don't have to have the same beans every day. There is such a variety of beans that you can have a different one each day. Pintos, black beans, white beans, split peas, red beans, lentils and black eye peas will give you a different variety each day of the week. With a pressure cooker you can cook them every day in just a few minutes. Soaking is not necessary but does shorten the cooking time and eliminates most of the gas causing sugars.

Corn bread is another staple that is on the menu each day. Nutritious, cheap and delicious, it goes great with beans and is easy to fix. Store whole dried corn and mix it with fresh ground wheat for a light textured wonderful bread. Ground cornmeal is on the list, but should be rotated every 6 months. Purchase powered eggs for the cornbread recipe.

Canned meats, such as chicken, tuna, and salmon will add needed protein and nutrients. Add whatever protein you like best. If you are a vegetarian, your own research will provide you with the necessary protein and nutrients.

Dinner Menus

Add beans and cornbread to each of these entrees.

Day one   Salmon patties or chicken patties

Day two   Chicken noodles

Day three   Spaghetti with sauce (with or without meat)

Day four   Chicken pasta Alfredo

Day five   Tuna or Chicken Casserole

Day six   Bean Soup with Chicken and Vegetables

Day Seven Black Beans and Rice with corn, salsa, tortillas. and cheese.

Recipes

Salmon Patties or Chicken Patties

1 can salmon or 16 oz can of chicken.

1 cup crushed crackers or dried bread crumbs

1 egg or powered egg equivalent

Vegetable oil for frying

Season with 1/2 teaspoon powdered garlic

Mix all ingredients together. Add oil to frying pan, about 1 tablespoon, more or less for your preference. Fry on medium high for about 3 minutes or until golden brown.

Serve with rice and beans.

You can add 1/4 cup of potato flakes to this recipe to give it more flavor and texture.

Chicken Noodles.

Cook noodles according to package (boiling them for about 10 minutes).

Add one can of chicken and 2 cups chicken stock

Add 1 cup milk

Add 1/2 teaspoon garlic powder

Salt to taste, about 1/2 to 1 teaspoon

Add Black Pepper to taste about 1/2 teaspoon

Add 1 tablespoon extra virgin olive oil

Simmer for about 5 to 10 minutes for the flavors to come together or as Emeril says, "so all the ingredients can get happy".

Serve with lentils.

Spaghetti with marinara sauce

Cook spaghetti according to package, or boil in 4 cups water for 8 minutes.

Add a little olive oil to keep spaghetti from sticking. Drain water from   cooked spaghetti.

Place spaghetti sauce in pan and warm

Add your favorite spices. I like lots of garlic and oregano.   Add dried Romano or parmesan cheese.

Serve on top of spaghetti or mix together

Serve with garlic toast and a side of white beans.

Chicken Pasta Alfredo

If you have alfredo sauce in a jar, this is real easy.

If not, here is the sauce recipe.

Add 2 tablespoons olive oil in a frying pan

Heat to medium

Add 1/4 cup flour a little at a time. It will brown in about one minute. Keep stirring it off the bottom of the pan. Then add 3 cups milk; stirring or whisking occasionally for about 3-5 minutes.

Add 3/4 cup dried parmesan cheese, whisking again.

Add 1/2 teaspoon or more of dried garlic

Add 1/2 teaspoon salt.

Serve over your favorite pasta. This meal is great with lentils or spit peas.

Tuna or Chicken Casserole

One large can tuna or two small 5 oz. cans

Dried mushrooms if you have them Soak them in   water for 15 minutes to rehydrate them.

 1 cup cheese If using dehydrated cheese, mix with water until it is thick like   syrup.

1/2 cup flour

2 tablespoons olive oil

Cooked peas, split peas or lentils

2 cups cooked rice

1 cup milk

1/2 teaspoon salt and 1/2 teaspoon garlic. black pepper to taste

Heat 2 tablespoons oil in frying pan. Add flour, stirring

until brown, about one minute. Add milk and whisk occasionally for about 3 minutes. Add garlic or garlic powder to taste.

In a casserole dish add all ingredients, mix well and bake for 20-30 minutes.

If you have dried onions, add them on top.

Bean Soup with Chicken and Vegetables

By this time you probably have some leftovers. You can add them all to this soup.

If not, it is great either way.

2 cans chicken stock

1 can chicken

1/4 cup flour

2 tablespoons oil

1 cup milk

Add your favorite mixture of cooked beans. The more different types you use, the better it is.

Add your favorite vegetables. Hopefully you will have some green beans and tomatoes.

Brown your flour in a frying pan with oil and add milk. Mix everything together in a large pot and simmer for 20-30 minutes. Serve with corn bread.

Here is another bean soup recipe you've got to try. Don't wait for a disaster to experience this great soup.

Perfect Bean Combination Soup

Beans – Lentils, black eyed peas, lima beans, black beans, split peas, white beans, pinto beans 6 cups total

Pre-soak beans overnight or at least 5 hours..

Change the water and rinse them well.

Place in pressure cooker, add 2 quarts water and cook at high pressure for 10 minutes.

Quickly reduce the pressure with cold running water and add the following ingredients.

½ teaspoon sea salt

2 tablespoons soy sauce

3 cloves garlic, minced

2 cups (16 oz) chicken or vegetable stock (No MSG)

1 jar (16 oz) tomato sauce or stewed tomatoes

Add more water (maybe just a few cups, your decision) and bring back up to high pressure and cook   5-10 minutes

Quickly release pressure and add the following.

1 chopped large onion'

1or 2 fresh ripe chopped tomatoes

2 tablespoons Italian seasoning. (should contain basil, marjoram, oregano, black pepper, rosemary and thyme)

Fresh ground pepper to taste

1 clove garlic

Bring back up to pressure and cook for 5 minutes.

Salt with soy sauce to taste.

This soup gets better with time. It is good in 20 minutes. It's great when it's heated up a second time. It is fabulous when heated up the third time.   Just wait, you'll see.

You will find that the lentils and split peas will disappear. It only takes a few minutes to cook them in a pressure cooker, and cooking for this length of time dissolves them. This is part of the reason this soup is so good. They form a thick gravy that has great flavor.

I cannot say enough about a pressure cooker. It is my number one kitchen tool.   There is more information on pressure cookers in Chapter Six.

Here are two desert recipes. You have all the ingredients for these on your grocery list.

Rice Pudding

¾ cup parboiled brown rice

2 cups milk

1/3 cup sugar

¼ teaspoon salt

1 tablespoon olive oil

2/3 cup raisins and ½ teaspoon vanilla extra will make a great addition but not necessary.

Cook rice according to directions. Add all other ingredients except ½ cup milk, egg and raisins and cook on low heat for 15 minutes. Add milk, egg and raisins and cook another 2-3 minutes, stirring constantly until thickened.

Serve warm. Delicious and nutritious.

Chocolate Brownies

1/2 c. butter or oil
4 tbsp. cocoa or 2 sq. chocolate
1 c. sugar
2 eggs, well beaten
3/4 c. flour
1/4 tsp. salt
1/2 tsp. baking powder
1 tsp. vanilla
1 c. nuts, chopped

Mix all ingredients together. Spread in well greased 9-inch square pan.

Bake at 350°F for 30-35 minutes. Let cool 10 minutes.

12 servings.

Most of us need to drink more water. It helps us lose weight, keeps our organs functioning well and flushes out toxins. It even prevents premature wrinkles

If you are like most Americans and drink a lot of bottled water, please change that unnecessary habit.

It is not just the fact that the plastic bottle is leaching chemical toxins into your water. Plastic bottles make up a large amount of waste in our landfills and our water systems. Do this for yourself and for your neighbors.

All you have to do is add a $15 filter to your faucet and buy a few stainless steel water bottles.

Great free healthy water with

no waste.

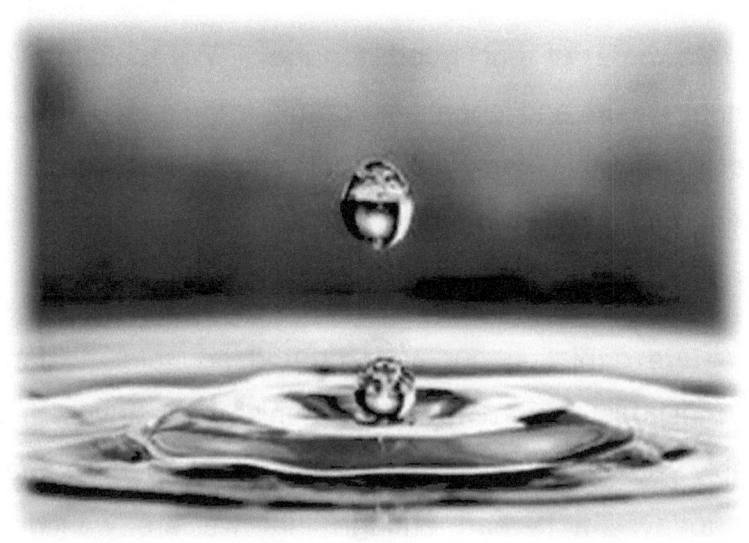

CHAPTER 4

Water

You can live for 3 weeks without food, but only 3 days without water. You will need at least one gallon per day per person in an emergency. More would be better. For a ninety day supply, you will need 180 gallons for two people. For this reason it is advisable to start planning *now*.

Water may possibly be the next big crisis in the world. In the United States we are so abundantly supplied with water that we have taken it for granted. We have not been very good stewards of our good fortune. We pollute it with industrial waste and chemical run-off from agriculture. We waste it irrigating farm land that should not be farmed, irrigating golf courses in the desert, and we allow raw sewage to seep into our rivers from our cities and towns.

We are depleting our underground aquifers at alarming rates, much faster than they can replenish themselves. This is probably the most irresponsible thing that modern man is doing today. It is bad enough that we are wasting our valuable resources such as our oil and gas reserves, but we can make it without them. It is bad enough that we are polluting the air we breathe, but we can deal with that, at least for the short term, but…

We cannot live without water.

And we still waste it like we have an unlimited supply.

Do you remember the drought we had in the Southeastern U.S. a few years ago? In 2007 the Southeast was hit with a drought that was scary. Many towns and cities were dangerously close to running out of water. Atlanta was less than 60 days from running out. Can you imagine the chaos that would occur in a city the size of Atlanta, if it ran out of potable water? The governor of Georgia was calling for people to pray for rain. I am all about praying, and I certainly see the benefits of praying for rain. But, don't you think the responsible thing to do would be to not waste the water in the first place?

That reminds me of a joke.

There was a flood and a very devout religious man prayed to be saved from the rising waters. Soon a boat arrived to take the man to safety. He refused to go, stating that God would save him. The water kept rising and another boat arrived. Again he refused to leave stating, "God will save me." The water kept rising and he had to get on to his roof to escape. A helicopter arrived to lift him off the roof, but again he refused to go, stating that God would save him.

Eventually the water rose over his house and the poor man drowned.

When he got to heaven, he asked God, "I prayed so hard, why didn't you save me?"

God replied, "What do you mean, I sent you two boats and a helicopter? What more did you expect?"

We have to help ourselves. God and Mother Earth have provided us with many wonderful resources, but it is our arrogance that has depleted these wonders with short sighted and selfish decisions. The Colorado River is a perfect example. We use it to supply water for cities, farms and golf courses in the desert. This huge and majestic river doesn't even make it to the ocean. By the time it reaches Mexico, it has been reduced to a trickle and eventually dries up. I have often wondered how karma might affect us with this selfish behavior. Don't you think the right thing to do is to let Mexico have some of this precious resource? Wouldn't that be the Christian thing to do, as in the Golden Rule? We seem to forget that our neighbors are our brothers, and we all are in the boat together.

Ok, I will get off my soap box and get to the point.

The point is that you need to take care of your water needs now.

Don't think you are in the clear because you have a well. Back in that drought in Atlanta a few years back, wells were going dry all around Georgia, Alabama, and the whole Southeastern United States. As the aquifers are depleted, so goes our wells. There is even discussion in certain states about regulating wells. You might see the local city or state government place a meter on your well, charge you for the water, and regulate how much you use. You may think it is your well and your property, but the water you take out of it affects your neighbor's well too. You can count on the fact that water will be tightly regulated in the near future.

It is pretty simple to collect rain water. You can make your house one huge water collecting machine. All you need is a water collection system and a big tank. The most complicated part is storing it. With your gutters piped to a tank, you can collect thousands of gallons of water in a few rain showers. Of course thousands of gallons of water require a large tank. If you can afford it, put in a 1500-3000 gallon underground septic tank to store this precious resource. It can irrigate your garden, flush your commodes, and provide you with refreshing water when you need it most.

There are less expensive means of storing water. You can purchase 200-300 gallon tanks available on the used market that sell for under $100. Make sure you know what was in it before you buy. I bought one that had a label for extra virgin olive oil. You certainly do not want one that stored chemicals.

One inch of rain will produce 600 gallons of water from a 1000 square foot roof. An easy way to figure how much water your roof will produce is to multiply the square footage of your roof by .6 gallons per inch of rain. If you have a 2,200 sq. ft. roof and ½ inch of rain, then the formula is …

2,200 x .6 x 1/2 inch of rain or 660 gallons of precious water to flush your toilets, water your garden or even drink, as long as you filter it or make sure you kill all of the bacteria in it. That's a lot of water for just a 1/2 inch of rain.

Here is another precaution. Several states make it illegal to collect rainwater without a permit. This is government at its worst. Apparently it is acceptable to spend our tax money and precious resources to clean and purify water, so we can flush our commodes. But, it is not ok to be good stewards of the water, store it and use it for our gardens. Go figure.

There are several ways to clean the water for use. A good filter is the best option. Your rainwater will not be pure to drink, but you can always filter it and purify it for your consumption.

Water Purification Systems

Everyone should have at least one purification system for your drinking water. The least expensive and easiest solution is a backpacker water filter. They cost as little as $20 and can save your life. Any sporting goods store will have them. The larger models for a whole house are important if you can afford them. The internet is an abundant source of information about water purification.

There are other easy and inexpensive ways to purify water in an emergency. Unscented common household bleach and hydrogen peroxide will work. Large filters are available at emergency food internet sites. You can make your own filters using parts that you can buy on the internet. All of these methods require thorough research, and this is a major area that you should become knowledgeable. I suggest that you purchase books or download information pertaining to this life saving system. Do not drink unfiltered or untreated water.

One gallon of water can be disinfected by 8-16 drops of regular household bleach (visually about 1/4 of a teaspoon). Double that for cloudy water. Shake and let the chlorinated water stand thirty minutes. One teaspoon will disinfect five gallons. Immediately after treating, water must initially have a slight smell of chlorine. If it does not, then repeat the process. Household bleach is relatively harmless in these tiny amounts. The smell of chlorine is not a bad sign. It indicates that water is treated and germ free. Once treated and disinfected, the chlorine smell will go away in a few days.

Regularly used water from large tanks may be treated once or twice a month with 1 Oz. bleach per 200 gallons or 5 Oz. bleach per 1000 gallons. Long-standing water in tanks can be disinfected with one pint household bleach per 1000 gallons. (2500 gallon tanks are fine with three pints.)

Bleach effectively kills bacteria and viruses, stops smells and then breaks down. Its effective germ killing alkaline property is completely neutralized very quickly. It does not stay chemically active in tanks for more than a few days. Most germs require sunlight to grow. Store water in the dark.

Make water a priority in your life. Give it the respect it deserves.

Here is a water story I found intriguing.

A man I knew from Upper State New York was having financial troubles in the bad economic climate in 2006. He went to the local university for advice. His business was failing, and he thought the professors could guide him. After some consultation, he was advised to relocate his business. The university's research concluded that the economy in that area would not be conducive to support his business for another 28 years.

He did just that, moved down south to North Carolina and is now very successful. He was still puzzled how these scientists and economists could come up with that 28 year measurement. He inquired of them again and asked about why it would take 28 years for the economy to get better in Upper New York.

The answer was water.

The university research showed that in 28 years, most of the country will be having a severe water crisis due to misuse and over use. Upper New York has an abundance of fresh water, and will be the place of choice for many people and businesses. Until then, the South will be growing with more people and businesses because of the mild climate. When the water crisis hits the South, the West and the rest of the country, the Northeast will be the new place of growth.

Water is going to be a big issue. Cities and states are fighting over it *now*. Take care of your water situation *now* so you will be prepared when the time comes.

Want a healthy snack? Your fresh whole grain bread could be the best solution.

It fills you up while providing healthy fiber to help you get rid of toxins. When you get rid of toxins, your immune system not only keeps you healthy, but helps you maintain your ideal weight.

A piece of whole grain bread drizzled with a little olive oil and balsamic vinegar is hard to beat. For a dessert, try whole grain toast with cinnamon and honey.

If you want a more filling spread, make a paste of leftover white or black beans. Add basil and garlic for a healthy low calorie snack.

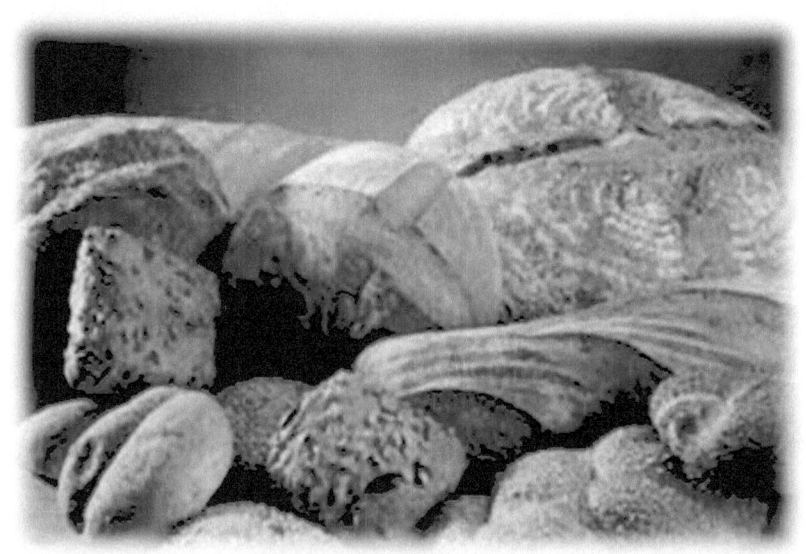

Chapter 5

Making Bread

Making your own bread is one of the most rewarding things you can do and is a crucial part of this preparation program. And to top it off, it is easy and takes very little of your time.

I love bread, and I suspect you do too. Bread is one of the most versatile foods. It provides good healthy calories and goes with everything you can put on a table. Nutritionally it can be fabulous, providing you with fiber, vitamins and minerals. On the other hand, it can also be totally worthless if made from white flour, white sugar and preservatives. This chapter focuses on the nutritious variety, using fresh whole grains and adding nuts and seeds.

There are many ways to make bread, and I hope you will experiment and discover what type you enjoy the most. For the purpose of this book, I am only going to focus on the easy way.

My source for this method comes from the book <u>Healthy Bread in Five Minutes a Day</u> by Jeff Hertzberg, M.D., and Zoe Francois.

I suggest that you purchase their book and experiment with the many types of bread they suggest. This is a great place to get started because making bread their way is easy.

I am providing my own adaption of their method. Get started, and you will be making good bread quickly. This is the "benefits you now" part while you get prepared for the future. Not only is this bread delicious and nutritious, it is inexpensive. A one pound loaf cost less than 50 cents, including the energy to make it.

You will be mixing enough dough to make four 1 lb loaves, and it will keep in the refrigerator until you are ready to bake. Try this and see how you like it. It takes a little preparation, but if you go to the grocery store today, you will be eating your own bread tomorrow. The longer it stays in the refrigerator, the better it tastes. The reason for this is that it starts to take on that sourdough bread taste. The dough will keep up to 14 days in the refrigerator.

It is best to store whole grain which you will grind yourself. Start *now* by getting your grain grinder and grain. The bread is more nutritious when made from fresh ground grain. Flour loses much of its nutrients after a few days from being ground, and whole wheat flour acquires a slightly bitter taste after a few weeks. The bread will be much tastier with fresh ground flour. However, to get started *now*, start with flour from your grocery store.

I have modified a recipe that tastes great and is designed for the person who follows this preparation method. It is simple and will get you started. I suggest that you get the book and experiment with other types of bread. You can make great bread and pizza dough with this recipe.

Ingredients

3 cups whole wheat flour

2 cups brown rice flour or parboiled rice flour

1/2 cup flax seed meal

2 cups all-purpose unbleached flour

1 1/2 tablespoon active dry yeast

(I use the larger bulk bottles but 2 packets will work just as well)

1 1/2 tablespoons sea salt

1/4 cup vital wheat gluten

4 cups lukewarm water

(Will feel warm, not hot to the touch)

Cornmeal for pizza peel

If you don't have whole wheat or rice flour, you can use 100% unbleached white flour. Reduce the amount by ½ cup and you won't need the wheat gluten.

Note: A bread stone and a pizza peel are great for baking bread. They are not totally necessary, but you should get them. They are inexpensive and usually come in a box set. The pizza peel is a wooden paddle you use to slide the dough onto the stone.

Measure the ingredients carefully. Mix the dry ingredients first with a whisk. Then add the water all at once. Mix with a stiff spoon until all the dry ingredients are wet. I use my hands to make sure I get all of the flour mixed. Do not knead it or punch it down. You just mix it until it is completely mixed, and then let it remain in your mixing bowl. Leave it at room temperature so that it will rise for approximately one to two hours. Put a loose lid (not air tight) on it while it rises. It can rise for more than 2 hours with no problem, but an hour is usually fine. It will rise and then flatten a little.

Now you are ready to start making the bread, but it has to rise again. Pull out enough dough to make a ball about the size of a grapefruit. It will be sticky and will stick to your fingers. Sprinkle flour on the dough to make it easier to work with. After sprinkling the dough with flour, wash hands to get the sticky off. Add some more flour and it will be easy to form into a ball. Now elongate the ball into an oval. Don't worry about the bottom not being smooth, it will smooth out as it bakes. This process takes less than a minute. The quicker you do this the better, because if you work it longer you will release gas pockets which will cause the loaf to become dense.

Put the elongated dough ball on a pizza peel that you have dusted with cornmeal. Cornmeal has oil in it that helps you slide the dough ball onto the stone. Let this rise and set for forty five minutes at room temperature, or 1 1/2 hours if you are taking the dough from the refrigerator.

When you are thirty minutes from the rising time, put the stone on the middle rack and set your oven for 450 degrees. I leave my stone in the oven so it is always ready to use. You may want to check your oven temperature with an oven thermometer, which you can buy for a couple of bucks at the grocery store. Ovens can be off by over 75 degrees.

When that time is up, slide the loaf onto the stone with a quick jerk. Bake for thirty to thirty five minutes. When it is done, let it sit for two hours for best results. If you are like me, you won't wait and will start eating the bread immediately. Can't blame you for that. Put a little olive oil or butter on it and enjoy.

I can't emphasize enough that you should buy a good "how to" book and do your own experimenting. These two books are great, but I am sure others are good too.

Healthy Bread in Five Minutes a Day

Artisan Bread in Five Minutes a Day

by Jeff Hertzberg, M.D., and Zoe Francois.

When the bread gets near the 14-day limit in the refrigerator, it may not rise as it should. This dough is great for making pizza or crackers. You can make pizza from the fresh dough, too. Just roll it out flat on your pizza peel. If it shrinks back, let it set for 15 more minutes covered. When you get it like you want it, let it rise for about 30 to 45 minutes. Add your toppings, preheat your oven and bake at 450 degrees for 25 minutes. If you want crispier crust, pre-bake the dough for 8 minutes, and add your toppings. Bake for an additional 10-15 minutes. This makes a great pizza.

When you have mastered the easy art of making bread, it's time to impress your friends. Invite them over and serve some fresh-baked bread with butter.   An even better combination is to drizzle extra virgin olive oil on a plate and then pour spots of red wine vinegar. I use garlic infused red wine vinegar, which I make by placing a few garlic cloves in the vinegar. This is great dipping sauce for fresh bread. It is also healthy for you.

Your friends will be impressed. This is a great time to talk to them about storing food for themselves.

Although this bread is great, my favorite bread is sour-dough.   Making sour-dough bread involves keeping a yeast starter alive in a jar which requires daily attention.   Most people may not have the time or be home every day. In a crisis you will have plenty of time to take care of those things. You will want to be productive, and doing things like this will keep you healthy and active. A sour-dough starter will be valuable and could also be a nice barter item in a crisis. For these reasons, I suggest that you learn the art of making sour-dough bread and keeping a starter, if only for a while. That way you will be prepared and ready to make a positive contribution to your family and friends.   Good luck and enjoy your new skill.

A great tool to have in an emergency is a cordless drill. Many hand grain grinders are designed so that you can power them with a drill. Just take off the handle and use the drill to take the work out of grinding your grain for your bread or your beer making.

The lithium battery drills are best, but all types work well. Consider getting a combination kit with a drill, flashlight and saw.

It is important to pick up a solar powered charger too.

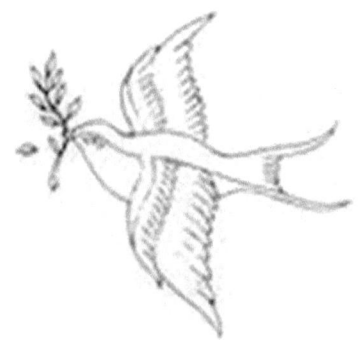

Chapter 6

Preparing Your Nest

Shelter is next in importance after food and water. In any kind of emergency expect that the electricity will be out for extended periods of time, and you need to be prepared. You are going to need heat and light. You will also need the ability to cook your food.

If you are fortunate enough to have extra money, concentrate on having a shelter far away from any city. Not everyone can afford this luxury, but if you have the resources, then do it. It is far more important to get your cabin in the woods than having cash in the bank or hoarding gold or silver.

In a major disaster crime can be rampant, especially in or around a city that already has a high population base. Make sure that your safe place has access to water. Creeks, streams and springs can be as good as gold in an emergency situation. They don't even necessarily have to be clean. You can always treat or boil your water.

Heat

If you live in a cold climate, you should prepare for some sort of heat. This is smart even if you live in a warm climate because weather patterns are changing.

Heating your shelter in the absence of electrical power is important, but more important is heating your body. The best and least expensive way to prepare for an emergency power outage in the winter time is to buy sleeping bags. Your house might be cold, but once you surround your body in a zero degree sleeping bag, you will warm up quickly. I sleep in a 20 degree sleeping bag. It keeps me comfortable, and I throw it on top of my bed. In the morning I toss it in the closet, and my bed is made, a lazy man's way of sleeping.

You should have one sleeping bag for each member of your household. They are not expensive. Not long ago, a zero or twenty degree bag would cost you over $100. *Now* you can find them at sporting goods stores for under fifty bucks. If you can't find a zero-degree bag in your price range, a twenty-degree bag will do. I have both, but I find that I can use the twenty-degree bag year round.

Now, you need to concentrate on heating your shelter. One of the best methods of heating your house in an emergency is a wood stove, if you live near a source of wood. In most areas of the United States where heat is needed, there are nearby forests. All forests have dead trees standing or laying on the ground, so you can get the fuel you need that is already dry and ready to burn efficiently. Of course you will need to have a chainsaw, an axe, splitting maul and wedges. Your chainsaw will need gas and oil to run, so storing those is necessary. Be sure to store gas conditioners because gasoline goes bad quickly, but can be prolonged with conditioners. There is a product called Sta-bil that you can buy at hardware and auto-parts stores. It will help stabilize your gas for long periods of time. One source on the internet said to use twice the recommended amount to store chainsaw gas for up to two years. Use metal cans, and store all combustible liquids in a safe place. You can also buy premixed chain saw gas that is stabilized. The label says it is good for 2 years. A few of those cans would be good to store.

If you don't know how to use a chainsaw, learn from an expert. Chainsaws are dangerous in the hands of a novice. Seek someone who repairs them or sells them, and ask for advice. You don't need a big powerful chainsaw, because you will be cutting mostly small trees and standing dead timber. A chainsaw with a fourteen or sixteen inch bar is a great choice.

A better choice may be to buy your firewood. In my area a pickup truck load of wood, already cut to size and split, is usually only $75-$100. There are other ways to creatively get your firewood. Used pallets are free in most any areas. Pallets can be cut up with a skill saw and will provide plenty of starter wood. I see free firewood available on the free section of Craigslist. Often the wood is sawed to length and just needs to be hauled home and split.

Propane is another source of emergency heat. It is more costly than wood, but is easy to store and much easier to handle than wood. Propane gas does not deteriorate, like other fuels such as kerosene. You can pick up portable heaters that attach to twenty pound tanks for under $80. A more permanent solution is to get a larger tank and hook it to a small wall heater. Hire a professional to do the piping. This is a sensible and inexpensive way to prepare for a power outage in the winter.

Heed this warning on all combustible heating systems. They produce carbon monoxide and require thorough knowledge of how they should be ventilated. Do your research, and know all about this potentially deadly combination. I prefer a vented wall heater that uses outside air for the combustion.

After you have provided an emergency source of heat, concentrate on making your house more energy efficient. Making your house more air tight is the most efficient way to start. Insulating a house does almost nothing to keep a house warm if there are drafts, and most houses have drafts. Unless your house has foam insulation, it is being bombarded with outside air that will get into the interior of your house. Start by caulking windows and doors, seal electrical outlets and look for all avenues of air infiltration. A handy device to give you feedback on temperature fluctuations in your house is a laser thermometer. You can point the laser at surfaces, and it will show the temperature of that surface. This is good for spotting air leakage and cold spots. These are typically very expensive, but a reliable and inexpensive version can be purchased from Harbor Freight Tools for under 30 bucks, or buy one on line at www.harborfreight.com.

Adding insulation is the next progression. Fiberglass insulation, in my opinion, is almost worthless. Wool, cotton and cellulose insulation perform better, especially when installed overhead. It is better to concentrate on putting more insulation overhead than in the walls or under the house. After all, heat rises, and you want to stop it from rising out of the house. All these types of insulation lose performance as the weather gets colder. Fiberglass insulation loses over half its performance value at 10 degrees Fahrenheit. When you need it most, like a thief in the night, it disappears. Foam insulation is the best and does not leave you when it gets cold. Foam is hard to retrofit and is usually only used in new construction.

Passive Solar Design

You can get an amazing amount of heat from the sun to help heat your house. Passive solar design can be as easy as enclosing a south-facing porch with sliding glass doors, or you can make your own small solar window boxes for less than the cost of a night on the town.

I enclosed my porch with used sliding glass doors and receive a lot of heat from it. It also acts as my greenhouse, starting plants and keeping year round plants. This was very inexpensive because I picked up the four sliding glass doors that I needed for this project for free. Craigslist is a wonderful thing. They even came with screens, so in the summer we enjoy a screened porch. This worked out well for me because my porch faces south. The only way you will get positive heat gain from any passive solar heating system is from a south-facing wall.

Mother Earth News has plans you can purchase for passive solar window boxes. You can do this yourself. If you scrounge materials, such as old storm windows and doors for the glass, you can build these practically for free. This magazine is a great resource for nearly everything you will need for a more sustainable lifestyle. I suggest you start getting current copies. Back copies make a great reference library.

You may also want to consider setting up a solar hot water system. Hot water is a luxury that we take for granted. In the event of a power outage if your hot water heater is electric, those warm showers will be missed. A gas water heater is a better choice and you can supplement either with solar. Solar water heating panels are not expensive, compared to solar panels that provide electricity, and you can usually find them used.

There are still quite a few panels left from the Jimmy Carter days, when he tried in vain to lessen our dependency on oil. A lot of people got them back then; but as the oil crisis lessened, they took them off their houses. They are out there, and you can find them with a craigslist search. I use searchtempest.com and search an area of several hundred miles. They are almost always for sale for around $200 each, new ones being nearly $800 each. A solar assisted water heater uses a small pump, powered by a small photovotaic solar panel, that circulates an antifreeze solution through a heat exchanger. This pre-heats your water and in many cases will provide all the hot water you need.

You can find do-it-yourself plans on the internet. Mother Earth News is an excellent source for information on solar designs. If you can afford to pay a solar company to put in a system for you, by all means do so. It will eventually pay for itself in good times and will be very valuable in an emergency situation.

Light

Unless you want to go to bed at 6:30 pm in the wintertime, you should plan for a source of light. Candles and flashlights are your first priority.

Flashlights are cheap and better than ever, especially the LED ones. They are so cheap that you should buy lots of them. Harbor Freight Tools occasionally sends out a coupon book with a coupon for a free flashlight. LED lights use a fraction of the battery power of conventional battery lights. You can get a good LED flashlight for under $5.

Don't forget to stock up on batteries. Batteries stored correctly can last for years. If you vacuum seal them and put them in your refrigerator, they will last up to 10 years. Count on them lasting a few years in your basement or a cool, dry dark place. Rechargeable batteries are great to have, if you have a solar battery charger. Harbor Freight Tools carries them along with solar battery chargers.

Another great and inexpensive light source is a solar outdoor landscape light. I just received this tip on an email. The person who sent it said that when the lights go out, they bring in their solar lights, put them in a drink bottle weighted down with sand and place them in each room. Probably won't give you reading light, but will certainly light up your bathroom.

Candles

Just like food, candles can be organic and good for you, or they can be laden with chemicals and not so good for you. Nearly every candle available in most stores is made from paraffin, a by-product of petroleum. Nearly every by-product of petroleum is dangerous to your health, especially if it is burned and you breathe the fumes.

Beeswax candles are your better choice. These candles produce less soot than their petroleum cousins and have a naturally sweet smell. Many claim that beeswax candles produce negative ions when burned, which cleans the air like an ionic air cleaner. These negative ions make you feel good and relaxed like being near large bodies of water. Some believe that one of the reasons the coast attracts so many people is because the ocean produces huge amounts of negative ions. Waterfalls are another source of negative ions.

Although they are more expensive, beeswax candles burn longer. They can burn 2 to 3 times longer than paraffin candles, so the true cost is not much different. Votives make a good choice. They are easy to place in a cup or a plate. They are also economical and burn more efficiently than larger candles.

Now would be a good time to take up a new hobby... candle making. It is really easy. You just need the proper equipment, which is very inexpensive. You can do it with a camping stove or microwave oven, glass measuring cup, a few molds, some wicks and some wax. This is one of those synergistic decisions that benefits you in the present and prepares you in the event of an emergency. Beeswax in bulk can be bought for around $10 per pound, and a pound can make a lot of candles.

You can sell beeswax candles to your friends and neighbors. Everyone needs to start preparing, and you could help them out. With a little boost from the internet, you could sell lots of them. In the event of a major emergency, you will not only be prepared, you will have another strong barter item. There is plenty of information on the internet to help you get started. YouTube.com is a great resource. You can spend hours looking at free instructions on how to get started.

After getting your candles, you might want to consider a

few electricity producing solar panels. It is getting easier to do this yourself, without having to hire consultants. It is also getting cheaper.

If you have the money, hire a good company and get set up with a solar emergency panel system to light your home. You can also run small appliances such as your grain mill with these free sources of energy. I recommend a system with a battery back-up, because there could be weeks of clouds and rain.

Again Harbor Freight Tools has a very inexpensive 45-watt solar panel system that you can install yourself. The price is usually around $200. Many times it goes on sale, or you can get a 20% discount coupon to bring the price down. You will need to add a battery to it, but generally it can provide you with 45 watts of lighting power that will greatly enhance your candle power. The new energy efficient light bulbs consume only 13 watts of power for the equivalent of 60 watts of traditional lighting. This small system can power up to 4 light bulbs in an emergency, (with a battery backup) which might be the ticket for enhancing your night life in a prolonged power outage.

Generators have come down in price and small ones can be bought for just a few hundred dollars. It would be best to buy one that is powered by propane considering that propane stores so well and gasoline does not. Generators are not good for running all the time, because they use a lot of fuel. I would only consider a generator to power large power items like water pumps, if you have a well.

If you have a hybrid car, you can make a few modifications and turn it into a generator. A simple method is to tie in a 750 watt inverter to your small battery. The hybrids turn off when the battery is charged so you won't be using fuel to run the car continuously. This will work for small appliances and lights. For larger users of electricity, you would want to do a more complicated modification. Google it and you will get lots of how-to information. I read where a Prius owner can power his whole house in an outage.

Cooking

The best cooking source is propane gas. A propane stove and oven can be your best friend in a power outage. If you have natural gas, which is much cheaper, stick with it. Chances are good that even in an electricity outage, the underground gas pipes might still be operational. However, to be prepared, buy a converter kit to change to propane in case you need it. Make sure you have a few propane tanks filled and ready.

If you can't afford to make that kind of investment, a small propane stove will work well. Camping stoves will work fine, but you should consider one that plugs into a 20 lb. or larger tank. Most sporting goods stores will have them. You will need a tank and a regulator. It will be important to purchase several tanks and have them filled.

If you have a gas grill, that might be just what you need, especially if it has a side burner on it. You can even bake bread in the grill part. Make sure you have a thermometer. Many recipes call for precise temperature measurement.

Pressure Cooker

Another must have appliance is a pressure cooker. Your grandma knew the benefits of this cooking tool, but it lost its luster with the advent of microwave ovens. It is really a shame that the pressure cooker is no longer used by more people. It actually cooks faster than a microwave, makes food taste better, uses less energy to cook and preserves the nutrients in food better than normal cooking or microwave cooking. You can take a lean, cheap piece of meat, such as round roast, and make it tender and delicious in a pressure cooker in less than 30 minutes.

Dried beans cook exceptionally fast in a pressure cooker. If you soak them overnight, most dried beans will cook in a pressure cooker in 6 to 8 minutes. I find that remarkable, since it takes an hour to cook them the usual way. You can cook small potatoes in 3 minutes, less time than it takes to cook them in a microwave oven.

The greatest thing about a pressure cooker is that you can cook an entire meal for a family of 4 in less than 20 minutes.

Don't believe me? Try this one pot meal.

Place parboiled brown rice, 2 cups, in the bottom of the cooker and cover with water to about 1/2 inch over the rice. Add 1 teaspoon salt. Use a trivet or another small pan with legs, (a folding steamer will work) and place 4 lean pork chops, separated from each other. On top of that, use another trivet and add fresh green beans. Don't cut up the beans, leave them long. Add slices of fresh red pepper for flavor, nutrition and color, and place in the trivet with the green beans. Add 10 to 12 small whole red potatoes with peelings on top of them. Top all of it with 3 fresh or frozen ears of corn, cut in half.

Bring the cooker up to pressure (takes about 5 minutes), and then turn the heat to low medium. Cook at high pressure for 10-15 more minutes. Let the pressure go down on its own, or quick-release the pressure by running cold water over your pressure cooker. Voila, you are done.

You will be amazed at how delicious this meal is that you

cooked it in just 20 minutes.   And you only have one pot to clean.

Isn't it crazy how we have bought into the propaganda and hype of new technology, when we had better technology right in our grasp? One of the reasons that pressure cookers fell out of favor is that the old ones were considered dangerous if you didn't use them correctly.   The new generation of pressure cookers has eliminated that concern by adding three safety valves. The old ones only had one. They even cook faster now.

My recommendation is that you purchase a stainless steel pressure cooker. The cheap ones are made of aluminum.   I do not cook in anything but stainless steel, copper or cast iron.

I bought my pressure cooker used on Ebay for $50. I did a lot of research and chose a Magefessa. It is excellent quality and made in Spain.   I think the new price is around $130. I received two pots with one lid. I use the smaller one the most since I am usually only cooking for one or two and use the large one when I cook a large one pot meal.

When you purchase your pressure cooker, also buy a good pressure cooker cookbook. You can find them on the internet. Then experiment. You will be amazed at the many things you can do with your new cooking tool.

There are several other areas that you should consider when preparing your nest.

Transportation is critical. If you live in the city, when it is time to get out, you will find the major routes have become a parking lot. You should study all escape routes should it become necessary to leave in the middle of a crisis. An older motorcycle, one that does not use computers or electronic ignition would be a good thing to have. My personal choice is a Kawasaki KLR650. You can purchase used ones for $1500. New ones are under $6,000. They come with their own risk, but can maneuver around traffic jams and can even travel off road.

Many of you will want to add guns and ammunition to your nest. This is a personal choice. If you feel that you will need a gun for protection, get one. The best gun for protection is a shotgun. All guns are dangerous, especially the automatic pistols. Make sure you know everything there is to know about the guns you choose to own, and get proficient with them. Safety courses are a must for a novice. I hear people talk about getting assault rifles, machine guns, even explosives. If you think that it will be necessary to go to those extremes, then you should carefully consider moving to a safer area, away from the high populated cities.

Communication will be critical. You will certainly want to know what is going on in the outside world. Cell phones and computers will probably be useless. A battery powered AM/FM radio is a must. One that cranks to charge the battery would be best. I suggest you have several for back up.

A ham radio operator will be in demand. This is a great barter idea. It is also something that you could take up as a hobby. Radio waves may be the only way we will be able to communicate with others in a disaster. Ham radios can communicate across the country and across the world. There are simple ways to get started and different levels of licenses. The beginning technician license is not that hard to get. It is free and you only have to pass an exam. The American Radio Relay League (ARRL) has a study manual for this purpose.

Housing

If you can afford to build a house, build a strong one. We are seeing weather patterns like we have never seen before... tornadoes in parts of the country that have never had them before, hurricanes with more force occurring more frequently, and earthquakes happening more frequently. The standard stick-built house of yesterday, (and unfortunately still being built today) can't stand up to these extreme weather forces. When houses are torn to shreds in a tornado and people are injured or die, it is because of inferior construction. Stick-built houses are inadequate and should not be built in the future. If you are smart, you will build with concrete.

My friend, Mark Barker, developed a new construction method using concrete, foam and steel. This is the house of the future. These houses will withstand almost anything that nature throws at it. They will not burn, will not mold, will not rot, are impervious to termites and can withstand over 200mph winds. They are green and extremely energy efficient. Many of them have roof patios, which is a great place for privacy, watching the stars and a small garden. And to make this even more incredible, they are just as inexpensive to build as a cheap stick built house. You can find out more about them at ***sumhouse.org.***

Heavy timber construction is another strong method of building. Timber frame structures have been around for centuries. The Germans perfected them in the past 200 years, but the Asians have built them for over 1000 years. There is one timber frame structure in China that is over 2,000 years old and is still in use. You can investigate these structures at ***mountaingreenbuilders.com.***

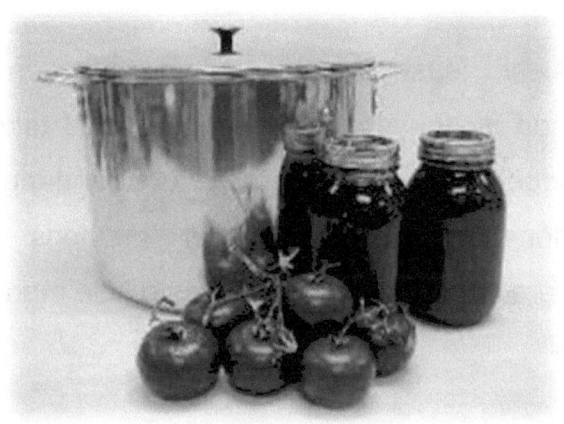

Chapter 7

Preserving Food

It's amazing to me the number of important things we have forgotten in this very recent span of history. For thousands of years preserving food has kept mankind alive. It was one of the most important skills that everyone knew and took part in. It was crucial for survival. Families survived the cold winters, because they had a large stockpile of preserved foods which provided them with valuable nutrition. The last generation to experience home preserving of food was the baby boomers. Today most people don't have a clue as to what it takes to preserve food, much less do it themselves. Fortunately it is easy and doesn't take a lot of retraining to learn this important skill.

The easiest, least expensive and safest method of preserving food is dehydrating. Canning food takes a little more knowledge and skill and can be not only dangerous but deadly if done incorrectly. Other methods such as fermentation are typically easy, just takes a little more work.

Dehydrating Food

Dehydrating food is the oldest method of preserving food. Our ancestors dried corn, vegetables, and meat with the sun. Jerky has kept many a traveler alive because it was lightweight, easy to carry and provided powerful calories that didn't require cooking. Utilizing the sun to dry foods costs nothing and takes very little work.

Drying food is easier, takes less energy and takes up less space than any other type of food preservation. The amount of tomatoes to provide four quarts of canned tomatoes can be dehydrated in one quart. Dehydrating doesn't require new seals each year like canning. A food dehydrator is basically all you need.

Any food can be dehydrated. Soups can be dehydrated

into leathers, flat sheets of preserved foods that have the appearance of fruit roll-ups. These leathers can be rehydrated into delicious soup. Leftovers can be dehydrated together, providing a full meal for a future date. Apples and fruits taste like candy when they are dried. They also make great desserts such as fried apple pies. Since the sugars are concentrated, these desserts require very little, if any, extra sugar. There is no limit to what you can do with dehydrating food. Of course, if you grow your own food, dehydrating can be a great way to store the excess bounty of food that gardeners have. If you don't grow your own food, you can buy end of season food at greatly reduced prices and dry them for practically nothing. We have a tomato farm near us, and every year at the end of the season they sell "pick your own" tomatoes for $5 per five gallon bucket. This totals twenty five pounds of vine ripened tomatoes for only twenty cents a pound. That's a lot of spaghetti sauce or pizza toppings.

I used my dehydrator to provide cheap meals for my son, Grayson, when he spent six months hiking the Appalachian Trail. I made organic nutritious meals for him that cost pennies, without preservatives. The commercial pre-packaged dehydrated foods cost as much as $5 per meal. Sometimes I would provide him with dehydrated nutritional supplements to add to Ramen noodles like dried mushrooms, dried tomatoes, dried broccoli, dried green beans, dried zucchini and dried hamburger.   Anything I could get for a bargain at the produce stand or grocery store went into his meals.

Electric dehydrators are inexpensive starting at around $20. I bought a dehydrator on eBay for $150. The round types are less expensive, hold less and are a little more difficult to handle. I prefer the square type with pull out trays. There are all types and brands. They are all very simple with a heating element and a fan. The less expensive ones seem to be as good as the higher priced brands. You will have to decide that for yourself. Do your research and get yours, so you can get started *now*.

Most foods take quite a while to dehydrate, some more than eight hours. I get my veggies ready and put them in the dehydrator at night so they would be ready the next morning. Be creative with your dehydrating, and you will be amazed at the amount of food you can store for very little money. Over ripe bananas are great to dehydrate and taste much better than the dried bananas you buy at the store. I encourage you to purchase some books to help you along with your own creativity.

One of my favorites is, Food Drying with Attitude by Mary T. Bell. She gets very creative and will open your mind about what all can be and should be dried.   Another good book that helped me was <u>Backpack Gourmet</u> by Linda Frederick Yaffe. She offers some great recipes like white bean pate` that are cheap and easy to prepare.

<u>Mother Earth News</u> is another great resource on dehydrating. There are plans available to make your own solar dehydrators, some out of cardboard boxes and aluminum foil. Foods dehydrated in the sun are more nutritious and contain vitamin D, a valuable vitamin during the winter months. A search on their website will bring up lots of information.

If you dehydrate foods with an electric dehydrator, set them out in the sun for a few hours after they are dry. They will pick up the vitamin D from the sun and will be much more nutritious.

Canning

Canning takes a little more effort but should be a part of everyone's food-storing package. Most all foods can be canned, but I prefer to can the high acid ones like tomatoes. These can be canned in a water bath canner, one that you can buy at any hardware store for under thirty bucks. You can preserve some great natural spaghetti sauces and salsas with your own special spices for pennies a jar. Other great high acid foods that you can preserve with your water bath canner are vinegar based pickles and chow-chow. Chow-chow with pinto beans makes a great and nutritious meal. Fruit preserves make great desserts.

If you are intent on canning low-acid vegetables like green beans, you should buy a pressure canner. They are not too expensive, usually under $100, and an aluminum one will work fine. I would not recommend a water bath canner because of the possibility of botulism, which can kill you. Canning done correctly in a pressure canner eliminates that possibility. With a pressure canner you can also preserve meats safely, too.

Again, I recommend buying a few good books to help you with this process. Even if you are an expert at canning, you will learn something new.

Other Food Preserving Methods

Fermentation is another great method. Sauerkraut comes to mind as the best addition to a great meal preserved by fermentation. There are many other types such as the highly nutritious oriental kimchi. Other foods including, tempeh, would be worth doing the research and adding to your diet, especially if you are a vegetarian.

Smoking meats and salting are other areas of preserving foods that may be worth your consideration. I find that these are too complicated for most people, but your research may prove me wrong.

Vacuum Sealer

A vacuum sealer will help you protect your dry preserved foods for the long term. Oxygen and light are the enemies of preserved foods. The vacuum sealer will seal out the oxygen and in most cases keeps the critters out. These are pretty simple machines. I suggest that you research on the internet and purchase one designed for commercial use. These will handle frequent use and will accept larger bags. I have found that the bags available for the commercial units can be less expensive bought in bulk on the internet. I bought a DZ280/A model from Sorbent Systems at www. sorbentsystems.com. I am happy with it, but encourage you to do your own research.

The mylar bags are best, but I find that most all heavy duty bags will work fine. You still may want to add an oxygen absorber to the sealed bags.

The bottom line is that food preservation is a skill everyone should know and should practice. It gets you in touch with your food just like growing your own food. It provides you with inexpensive natural food without preservatives today and will enhance your food storage system for tomorrow. This type of skill gives you the confidence to prepare you for anything that the future holds.

.

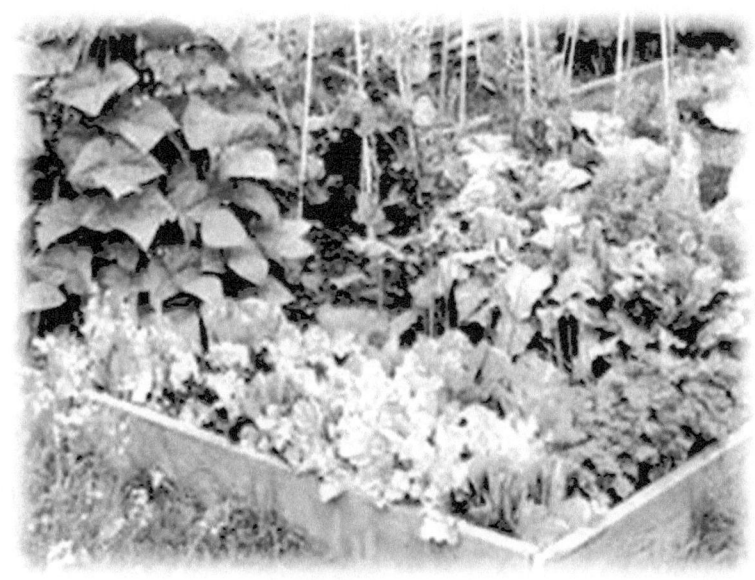

Chapter 8

Grow Your Own Food

Growing your own food is not hard. As a matter of fact, it is rather easy and very satisfying. You don't need to grow everything, just the things that are most practical and most nutritious.

Everyone should eat some raw fruit and vegetables every day. Only raw food contains live enzymes that aid in our health and protect us against disease. The heat of cooking depletes vitamins, damages proteins and fats and destroys enzymes which benefit digestion. Raw food has the best balance of water, fiber and nutrients. Cooking also creates free radicals in food. Lower your amount of free radicals and you will lower your chances of disease and premature aging. I am not advocating giving up cooking, because that is not necessary. It is just important to eat some raw foods every day.

The best way to include raw food in your daily diet *now* and in the event of a disaster is to grow your own. You can easily grow lettuce indoors or in a sun-room. Salads are the easiest way to get raw foods in your diet, and most salad items are easily grown. Many salad items such as spinach and kale can grow year-round in most areas of the United States. Crops such as broccoli and cabbage grow until the climate gets very cold, and then they store easily in a cellar or in the earth itself.

When considering what to grow, let history be your guide. There are certain foods that have kept mankind alive for centuries and should merit your consideration. These foods are not only nutritious; they also store well. Foods such as cabbage and potatoes are highly nutritious and will store all winter and spring until the next crops come in. Before the potato famine, the Irish ate a diet of mainly potatoes, milk, barley and beans. Greens of all kinds are easy to grow.

My mother-in-law grew up in Bryson City, North Carolina, a once poor mountain community, in a time when you had to provide your own food. She told me that her family grew lots of cabbage and potatoes, and many times that is all they had to eat. At the end of the fall harvest, they would pull up the cabbage, root and all, and then bury the cabbage head right there in the ground, where the roots were. Then they covered it over with soil and leaves.

"On many occasions, I had to go outside and get a cabbage. I'd uncover the snow, dig it out and bring it to the table. We ate fresh and delicious cabbage throughout the winter. Nothing's better with beans and corn-bread"

... Minnie Bartlettt

Cabbage and potatoes are easy to grow and should be on the top of your list for a fall crop to prepare for winter.

Growing Vegetables Outside

My method of organic growing came from Mother Earth News. There are thousands of books that will guide you in your pursuit of growing vegetables. Mother Earth News magazine is one of the best sources for the home gardener, especially the organic gardener. Their website, www.motherearthnews.com, contains a mountain of information that is invaluable to the home gardener. I highly recommend subscribing to this wonderful resource and even buying back issues. The Guide to Growing Food, spring 2010, is a must have.

Organic gardening is easier and more fool proof than chemical gardening. With chemical gardening, it is difficult to get the right nutrient combination to allow the plant to grow at its maximum level. It can be tricky to make sure you have enough fertilizer without giving it too much. Adding too much nitrogen is worse for the plants than adding no nitrogen at all. The chemical fertilizers are just too powerful to regulate easily. And of course who wants chemicals in their food anyway?

I discovered this method of gardening in that spring 2010 issue. When I tried it, I was amazed at the ease of use and the quality of plants it produced. I only had to fertilize once at the beginning of the planting for low demand vegetables. For higher demand ones, a second application is all you usually need. I didn't do anything else, except water the plants.

This fertilizer recipe came from Mother Earth News in an article written by Steve Solomon. I suggest you purchase Steve Solomon's books. He has been doing this with a passion for over thirty years, and his books are wonderful resources. A former school teacher, Steve still has the passion to teach and help others grow great vegetables. You can purchase his book, Gardening When It Counts from the

<u>Mother Earth News</u> website for $19.95.

Another must have resource is the back issue DVD from Mother Earth News, from 1970-2010. There are articles covering subjects from building your own house to building solar collectors to home gardening. This magazine is for the do-it-yourselfer and will be a valuable resource for you in the present and in an emergency.

Organic Fertilizer Recipe

4 parts seed meal. Soybean meal is probably the cheapest, but any seed meal will work.

1/4 part agricultural lime, calcium carbonate

1/4 part gypsum (if you can't find it, double the agricultural lime)

1/2 part dolomitic lime (do not use hydrated lime)

1 part bone meal

1 part kelp meal or ground kelp

Purchase kelp meal in bulk on the internet or from an agriculture supply store. It is usually about $50 for a fifty pound bag, plus shipping. The small bags are expensive. I have seen them for $25 for a five pound bag.

Mix this up in a 5-gallon bucket, and you are ready to plant. How much do you use? Steve recommends the following proportions. In a raised bed garden, you can mix this in with your soil. Make sure you have plenty of compost mixed in with your soil to keep it light. Add a layer of composted manure on top. You can purchase compost, but if you are on a budget, leaves or sawdust will work well. Rotted sawdust is best but it doesn't have to be rotted. Just make sure the sawdust is not from walnut trees, which has a chemical that inhibits plant growth.

Low demand vegetables get four quarts fertilizer per 100 sq. ft. He recommends adding 1/4 inch layer of finished compost or composted manure. You can buy a bag of finished manure for less than two dollars. These plants include beans, kale, beets and turnip greens.

Medium demand vegetables get four to six quarts fertilizer per 100 sq. ft. plus 1/2 inch layer of compost or manure. Some medium demand plants are basil, cabbage, lettuce, potatoes, small peppers, spinach and zucchini.

High demand vegetables get four to six quarts fertilizer plus 1/2 inch layer of compost or manure. These include cantaloupe, Brussels sprouts and tomatoes.

High and medium demand vegetables will require side dressings of the fertilizer every few weeks. If you want to know more about which vegetable are high, low, or medium demand, check out the Mother Earth News website, and you can search for Steve Solomon's article. Or better yet, buy his book and have it for your reference.

Use this recipe, cover your ground with mulch to keep out weeds and keep in water. Water your plants regularly, and you will have an abundance of vegetables for you, your family and your neighbors.

Another inexpensive way to add organic fertilizer is to use manure. Rabbit manure is best in that is can be used directly on your garden and doesn't have to be aged or composted. It is balanced and has all three of the elements necessary for plant growth... nitrogen, potassium and phosphorus. It also has less odor than other manures. I purchase rabbit manure from a rabbit farm and pay $40 per truck load. That is plenty for most home gardens.

Other manures such as cow, chicken or horse should be composted first. Chicken manure has much more nitrogen that any other organic fertilizer. But beware that the smell could cause you problems with your neighbors.

I use a combination of manure and Steve Solomon's fertilizer recipe. That seems to give my plants a good balance and is not too costly. The successful organic gardener will use combinations of fertilizers and composted matter.

Another must have valuable resource is <u>Square Foot Gardening</u> by Mel Bartholomew. His research will provide you with a great space-saving way to garden. With his method you can grow more vegetables in less space with less work than any other type of gardening. With the use of vertical gardening, you can grow plenty of food for a family in a small space. It is a great way to get started in gardening. He even has a garden plan for children to help them get started. What better way to get children in touch with their food.

Vertical gardening is just starting to gain popularity. It is a must for the home gardener and especially the patio gardener. With vertical gardening you can grow twenty square feet of plants in just four square feet. There is an abundance of information on the web. Check it out and you will find an easy, space saving way to grow your own food. *Phytopods* out of California have a system ready for you to grow a variety of plants.

Easy Potato Vertical Growing Method

Try this easy and space saving way to grow potatoes. You grow them vertically in a cage. At harvest time you remove the cage and an abundance of potatoes fall to the ground.

Make a round wire cage about 3 to 4 feet in diameter. You can use chicken wire or any inexpensive wire fencing that comes in three to five foot widths. Chicken wire is the least expensive. Hog wire is more expensive but works great if you want to harvest new potatoes as they grow. The hog wire is spaced so that you can put your hand through the cage and harvest the potatoes. Tie the cage together with string or wire. Use a stake to hold the cage vertical.

Now you are ready to plant. Place about six inches of compost or topsoil in the bottom of the cage. Plant six to nine seed potatoes and cover with more soil or compost. You can use straw too. Soak it with water and wait a few weeks.

When the leaves are about 6 inches tall, cover them again with more compost or soil, leaving about two to three inches of leaves above. Wait a few more weeks and do it again. Keep this up until they are near the top. New potatoes will grow with each addition of soil. Wait until the leaves start to wither and you are ready to harvest. Harvesting is easy.

Before you try this, check out the videos of youtube. There are plenty, and they will give you more ideas as well. Be sure to add a little manure to your compost and you will be rewarded with a huge supply of potatoes for your table and for your food supply.

Water, Water, Water

No amount of fertilizer or compost will help a garden without water. Along with sunshine, it is essential. The problem most gardeners have is that they don't water enough. In the heat of the summer, you can expect to water every day.

This can be difficult and time-consuming. That is why I recommend drip irrigation. It makes the most common sense.

First of all, it conserves water. It slowly drips water at the plant's root zone, saving an estimated 50-75 % over sprinklers. Secondly, you will have fewer weeds, because you will not be watering the areas around the plants. In other words, you won't be watering your weeds. And finally, it is less work. After setting up the system, you only have to monitor it daily to make sure nothing gets clogged.

There are plenty of resources to help you with this. The internet is full of free advice, and, your local garden supplier can help you with everything you need.

You should be planning to collect rainwater from your roof. You will be surprised at how much rainwater you can collect from one day's rain. As a matter of fact, if you don't have a large container or containers to collect it, you will send more away than you will collect. Collecting rainwater will give you all the water you need for your garden if you plan it right and get a large enough container.

Indoor Gardening

Indoor gardening is pretty simple. You mainly need to use containers and grow the same way you do in your garden. Use the same fertilizer and soil… the lighter the soil the better.

A good soil mix is 1 part vermiculite, 1 part perlite, 1 part composted manure and 1 part potting soil. If that gets a little complicated, buy potting soil and add about 20% perlite or vermiculite to add water retention and drainage. To this mix you add about a cup of your organic fertilizer mix per plant.

Self-watering containers save labor and also prevent you from over-watering. They keep a constant supply of moisture to the plant, helping to reduce stress and help the plant grow better. You can buy them at most gardening stores, but you can easily make your own. On the Mother Earth News website, type "container gardening" in a search to get information for making containers using two five-gallon buckets. There is plenty of information on container gardening on this site. These containers can be used indoors or outdoors.

Light is extremely important for the indoor garden. You may have a greenhouse or sun-room, but you still might have to add more light. You don't even need a sun room, if you have the right light source. And you don't have to buy expensive grow lights. Inexpensive shop lights cost about

$10, and the bulbs are about $5 each.   Be sure to get the high intensity bulbs, about 6500K.   The small diameter bulbs, T- 5's are best, a little more expensive but worth it in the long run.   You will need to place these lights close to the plants and put them on a timer, with up to 18 hours of light per day.

Indoor growing stores are popping up all over the country. They host a wealth of information and will have everything you need to set up your indoor garden.

Vegetative plants are best to start with. By that I mean plants that do not have to flower or fruit. I recommend starting with leafy veggies such as romaine lettuce, kale or spinach. They can be grown with the less expensive fluorescent lights which require a lot less electricity than the more expensive high pressure sodium lights that flowering plants require.

Hydroponic and aeroponic methods are great ways to grow indoor plants. There are plenty of good but expensive systems available for you to get started quickly. If you are a do-it- yourselfer, you can check websites that teach indoor marijuana growing. The marijuana growers have gotten these methods down to a science, and a lot of their information is free on the internet. Try *stinkbuddies.com* for a complete method of growing indoor plants. This site gives you all the info you need to grow indoor plants, including how to inexpensively make the apparatus to easily disperse the nutrients and hold the plants. Even though this site is primarily for growing marijuana, you can grow good nutritious salad vegetables using these same techniques. Again if you are only growing vegetative plants like lettuce, you will not need the expensive grow lights.

Animals

Some of you may want to consider raising animals for food. It is much more involved but can be very rewarding. As part of my preparation and research for this book, I started raising chickens and pigs. What a learning experience! This is something that you should consider carefully because you could bite off more than you can chew.

Chickens are easy and should be your first experiment. I was interested in chickens for eggs, not for meat. It was pretty easy to keep 7 hens and one rooster. I let my chickens free-range, but you can only do that if you live in the country. Even then it is risky due to the predators that lurk, especially dogs. You don't need a rooster if you keep them in a coop. Roosters will protect the hens from certain predators. If you live in the city, you probably cannot have a rooster anyway. A few hens are easy to keep on a small lot. It is wise to prepare and store extra feed for them in an emergency. There are plenty of resources out there that can help you get started

Chickens may be easy. Pigs are not so easy. You really need to learn all about them before you start or you will end up like me, learning from the school of hard knocks. You don't want to get a phone call from your neighbors complaining that the pigs are rooting up their lawn. Pigs are little Houdini's and can escape the most well built pen. Pigs are good to have and could be your barter asset. They multiply like rabbits and are really not that difficult to keep if you have time and know what you are doing.

I would also consider sheep and goats, for the milk they produce. Goats can survive on very little grain food if you allow them to eat the weeds and brush that they love. Be careful though, they will eat your garden too if you do not contain them well.

Rabbits are easy to raise for food. When you raise animals for food, you get the added benefit of the manure fertilizer they produce. One of your best resources is the book, The Self Sufficient Life and How to Live It by John Seymour. It covers about everything you need to know about living a sustainable, self sufficient lifestyle.

One of the most interesting ways to grow your own food is aquaponics. This synergistic method produces several food crops at once. Fish is grown in a tank while vegetables are grown just below or beside the tank. Through the use of pumps, the fish fertilize the plants and the plants clean the water for the fish. There is even a method of attracting and harvesting the black soldier fly to feed the fish. It is fairly simple to set up your system with an old bathtub. For more information on this method, check out Murray Hallam's website at aquaponics.net.

Another easy way to produce food and barter items is to grow mushrooms. It is pretty simple and easy to do. Shitake mushrooms can be set up with a stack of logs, and the logs will produce mushrooms for eight years. For around twenty dollars and a ½ days work, you can have a bounty of annually producing mushrooms.

If you live in the country, consider honey bees. You can get honey and beeswax from your efforts, while enhancing your plant life around you. You may even be able to get a grant to start your honey bee venture. Honey bees have been dying at an alarming rate. No one has discovered the answer to this problem, but many suspect that it is due to the large amounts of pesticides and herbicides that are applied in our agricultural fields. Genetically modified plants may also play a role in that they produce a toxin in their skin that kills insects.

The government is very concerned and rightly so. Honey bees pollinate the vast majority of our crops, making them crucial to our food system. Having your own bees will help others while helping you.

There are plenty of other resources out there for you to research. Get started *now* and you will find that it is easier than you think.

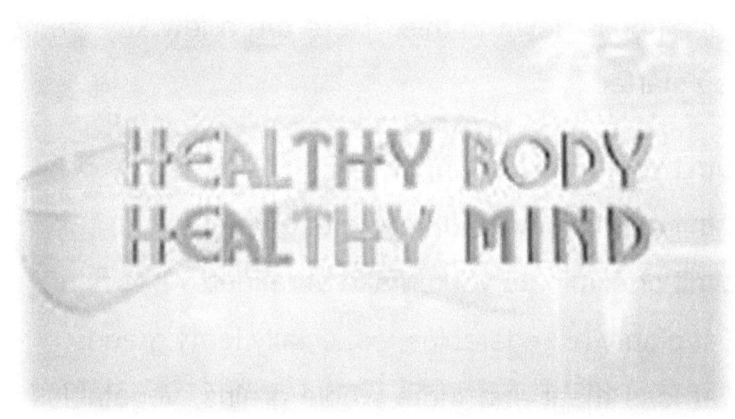

Chapter 9

Your Body

In the event of a major disaster there will be very limited access to medical aid. You will be best served if you are healthy. That is why you should prepare your body *now* to make it as healthy as you can. This is another one of those statements that I feel I must repeat.

You should prepare your body now to make it as healthy as you can.

There is plenty of information on the internet and in books to help you do this. I won't go into too much detail, but in a nutshell it all boils down to this. Here are a few key elements to get you started.

- Limit your intake of sugar.
- Limit or eliminate your intake of animal fats.
- Limit or eliminate your intake of refined white flour.
- Eat plenty of vegetables, especially leafy greens.
- Eat less meat and more whole grains, vegetables and fruits.
- Eat some raw fruits and vegetables every day, such as a salad with nuts and raw fruit.
- Choose good fats for your body such as extra virgin olive oil.
- Choose organic foods as often as you can.
- Eat lots of garlic.
- Eat dried beans on a regular basis.
- Eat oatmeal for breakfast with flax seeds, cinnamon and a little honey.
- Drink lots of clean water every day.
- Exercise your body every day. Walking is good.
- Relax and reduce stress.
- Chew your food well. This is the first stage of digestion.
- Maintain an active empowered mind

If you are taking medications, it would benefit you to research natural ways to get the same benefits. Visit a natural healer, and you will get a wealth of information.   I am not suggesting getting off those medicines. I am only advocating that you know alternatives should your medicine be hard to get. There are many natural remedies that have been used for thousands of years that are good. It is up to you to find them out for your own personal situation.

The Current Environmental Disaster

You should not only prepare your body for a possible future disaster; you should prepare your body now to fight off the current disaster. With a healthy immune system, you will be able to defend yourself against the multitude of things that attack our bodies on a daily basis today.

We have a tsunami of toxins attacking our immune systems and vital organs. It is happening *now* and has been going on for decades. This is the worst disaster that this country and the rest of the world have ever experienced. The problem is that no one really notices it. It has killed millions, is still killing millions and will continue to kill millions in the future. You cannot escape it. It is here, there and all around you.   It is the invisible disaster.

The people in Japan just got an extra dose of an

environmental disaster on a mega scale. No one knows the horrors of radiation sickness more than the Japanese. My heart goes out to them for having to experience this again

Many people believe that food allergies, cancers and most all sickness comes from the environment and the toxins that surround us... toxins that we breathe... toxins that we eat... toxins that we smear on our face and bodies.

Do your best to limit your exposure to as many toxins as you can, and protect your body naturally from toxins you cannot avoid. This can be as simple as avoiding foods wrapped in plastic or foods in cans. Canned food has a plastic liner that emits small amounts of toxins. I know you cannot avoid this altogether; as a matter of fact, canned foods make up a huge percentage of our food storage system. But you can avoid them *now* by buying and cooking fresh foods. The worst foods in cans are the highly acidic ones such as tomatoes and tomato sauce. The acid causes the toxins in the plastic liner to leach into the food. You can purchase them in jars, which are much better for your body. Buy spaghetti sauce and salsa in jars.

Serve fresh and naturally preserved foods. We have somehow been led to believe that fresh food is too difficult or time-consuming to fix. This is a myth. It's just as easy and quick to fix dried pinto beans in a pressure cooker as it is to open a can and heat it up. You can cook fresh greens beans easily as well. Almost anything you can get in a can, can be cooked fresh with very little effort. Fresh green beans take only 3 minutes to cook in a pressure cooker.

The best thing you can do to protect yourself is eat healthy foods and exercise. There are many natural remedies that can assist your immune system. Basil is thought to protect against radiation. Garlic acts as an antibiotic. Many herbs are thought to protect against many types of ills. It is up to you to find and use them for your best interests.

Great Herbs and Foods for Health

Parlsey   Rich in anti-oxidants and especially vitamin K Good for keeping the mouth fresh and keeping teeth healthy

Kelp   Many nutritional properties   Contains natural iodine making it good for the thyroid Has lots of anti-oxidant properties and used by the Japanese for protection of radiation exposure

Garlic   Used in Russia during World War Two as an antibiotic, they referred to it as the natural penicillin. Has many disease preventing and heart healthy properties Maybe more than any other herb

Basil   Great for vision and good for the skin   Known as a natural protector from radiation exposure

Oregano   Has anti-septic and antibiotic properties   Can be taken orally for colds and influenza

Maitake Mushrooms Cancer   preventative,   immune support, blood sugar control, lowering blood pressure, lowering cholesterol and weight management are just a few of the healthy properties of this amazing food. All mushrooms are good but Maitake is the best.

Ginger   Has   anti-inflamatory   and   anti-flatulent properties   Can prevent nausea due to motion sickness and pregnancy Also known to relieve migraine headaches

Turmeric   Anti-inflamatory and thought to be a cancer preventative   Also used as a medicine to prevent Alzheimer's disease

Cinnamon   Helps regulate blood sugar levels and protects against cell damage from free radicals   May also help in weight management

Rosemary   May cut cancer risk by cutting the carcinogenic compounds in cooked meat   Also known to help with yeast infections

Black pepper   Loaded with anti-oxidants, healthy for the skin and digestion   Helps with weight loss by breaking down fat cells

Mint   Can be used as a digestive aid and helping relieve   irritable bowel syndrome Also good for sore muscles and fresh breath   This perennial is very easy to grow and should be grown in containers, or it will take over your garden.

Cilantro or coriander   Provides lots of vitamins A and K Used in traditional medicine as a digestive aid and an aphrodisiac   Lowers the bad and increases the good cholesterol, making it a great healthy heart herb

Paprika   Paprika (dried red bell peppers) is inexpensive, full of vitamin C and has lots of anti-oxidant properties. Great healthy addition to add to any food

Sage   Known as the thinkers herb, has been associated with relieving depression   Provides essential oils Had numerous uses by Native Americans

Ancho Chili Powder   Great for heart health   Depresses appetite and increases metabolism Any hot pepper is good

Stevia   A great herb to grow, because it is a non carbohydrate sweetener, forty times sweeter than sugar   Has anti-biotic properties and may increase dental health

Lemon   Great for skin, preventing acne   Also prevents wrinkles, loaded with vitamins and anti-oxidants   Kills bacteria, good for a mouthwash

Tomato powder   Loaded with vitamins and minerals, especially lycopene, thought to prevent cancer, especially prostate cancer   Enhances colon health

Add these to your present diet and your food storage system. You will not only benefit from the immune system building properties, but they add wonderful flavor to food as well. Most of these can be bought in bulk for savings. Some of you will grow and dehydrate your own. These herbs will make you healthier and help feel better as well.

There are many natural ways to enhance your health. Start *now* by making a commitment to good health and discovering these wonderful and healthful remedies. The Chinese and Indians have been using natural means of health care for thousands of years and can lead you to your discovery of health. There are so many remedies and tips on the internet that it can be overwhelming. As stated earlier, use your intuition and let it guide you toward your health and happiness.

What we eat is only a part of our health. Stress is one of the most damaging causes of ill health. We take it for granted, and many people actually think that stress is just a natural part of our life. It is not, and you should start *now* by reducing stress in your life.

Start with the causes. It may take some introspection, a trip alone into the wilderness or a trip out of town to get in touch with your true advisor. That is the little voice of intuition that is inside all of us. It only speaks to us when we get quiet and listen. But it speaks our truth. It speaks to us to help us live a long, happy and healthy life. Let it guide you to a new you. You will be more relaxed and start enjoying every waking moment.

Reduction of stress doesn't mean the reduction of negative events that occur in our life. We will always be confronted with negative events. It is how we react to these events that affect our health.

Exercise is another important part of the good health equation. We don't have to go to the gym, nor do we have to exercise vigorously. We just need to move our muscles to keep them fit. Walking and slow jogging are probably the best forms of exercise. Not only does walking help your muscles and especially your heart, it helps you stay slim and relax. As you walk, repeat positive affirmations to yourself, reaffirming your joy in your life and in the universe.

Know that words and how you speak to yourself and others are very powerful. Pay attention to your words and phrases. Remove the negative ones. Add positive ones. For instance, instead of saying, "That just pisses me off," replace it with "That just burns my fat." Sometimes I hear people say, "That just makes me sick." If you say that or anything close to it, change it. You may or may not believe it, but words are powerful, and when repeated over and over again, can cause negative or positive events in your life.

Empower yourself.

When we have power, our bodies protect us in mysterious ways. When we lose power and feel helpless, our bodies begin to deteriorate. Psychologists have observed this for years. Have you ever noticed how some people work all their lives to retire, and soon after they do, their health suffers? This is due to a loss of power. When working, especially in powerful and important jobs, the confidence that is obtained is a strong protector of the immune system. When it is abruptly taken away, the body can suffer. Many retirees try to replace that power by volunteering, but it is not the same.

How can you empower yourself? Learn something new or take on a new challenge. This will not only empower you but will also stimulate your brain. Stimulating your brain is another excellent way to avoid brain disorders like Alzheimer's disease. As part of my preparation plan, I recently went back to school. This is the same school where I taught 30 years ago. It is amazing how empowering it is. And it is not easy. My plan was to learn some skills that I could use in an emergency, not only to help my preparation, but to enhance my barter skills as well. I enrolled in the technical program at McDowell Technical College in the maintenance technology program. Here I am getting proficient at electrical work, machining and welding. I had always thought that this type of technology was easy and less demanding than my four-year college degree. Boy was I wrong! I had to take Algebra and Trigonometry to prepare me for my electronics class. Even though I took it in college 35 years ago, it was very tough. I made an A but had to work hard for it. In class I felt young again, even though I was the oldest person in the class. The students treated me as one of them and didn't seem to notice the age difference. It felt good bonding with the other students as we discussed the upcoming test or collaborated on our homework. I even got a smiley face on one of my assignments, which I promptly put on my refrigerator. My electronics class, AC/DC technology, was the hardest course I have ever taken, giving me a new respect for technical college students. I also have a new respect for the empowerment you get by going back to school

Know that anything you can do to expand your mind will help your overall health. This is important in preparing your body and mind for anything that the future holds.

Give and Receive

It is a known fact that those who give to others receive the benefits of good health. A great way to do that, without costing you any money, is to give blood on a regular basis. You get a free mini check up (blood pressure, iron level) while giving yourself the opportunity to help others and save lives. That alone is enough to make you feel good about yourself to enhance your health. There are other reasons giving blood is healthy. For some, who have too much iron in their blood, it reduces the iron level. Another strange unknown reason, you just feel better after you give blood. I don't know whether it is because your body is refreshing and generating new blood, or if it is because you have helped others, but for some reason, the day after I give blood, I am flooded with endorphins. I get this euphoric natural high that I can't really describe. Try it. I think you'll like it.

It is your right and your destiny to be healthy, happy and joyful. Choose to be, and you will receive the benefits of great health and wellness. It may take some effort to make positive changes, but it will be worth it *now* and in the future.

Your Teeth

A lot of people put off their dental work until the last moment. In a disaster, you may not have that chance. *Now* is the time to take care of your dental problems. Dental work is expensive, and many people just can't afford it. There are alternatives, and you should explore them.

Two years ago I researched Costa Rica as an alternative. I needed over $10,000 worth of dental work and did not have the money to do it, even though I had dental insurance. I had heard of dental tourism but didn't pay it much attention. The $10,000 price tag gave me the incentive to check it out. I could not have been more surprised and pleased.

Basically I went to Costa Rica for a week, got the best dental care of my life and enjoyed exploring this beautiful country for $3,000, saving $7,000 in the process. Dental tourism is important to them, so they are good at what they do. I plan to go back this year to complete some more work, including implants. You can stay at hostels for an inexpensive price, (usually $10 per night) and meet people from all over the world. My favorite hostel was in Arenal, the Five Star Backpacker Hostel. With an amazing view of a volcano, it had a great pool and outdoor lounging area. While there for three days, I met people from 12 different countries. I look forward to going back.

Other countries have capitalized on medical tourism as well. Check out India if any type of surgery is in your future. The cost can be a fraction of the cost in the United States, including the airfare and hotel expenses. I have been told that the hospitals in India are immaculate and the care there is very good. One person on the internet said that he went there for heart surgery. The reported total cost including airfare and hotels was under $20,000.

In conclusion, I want to emphasize that health is your duty. It is your duty to yourself and to others. We have the greatest health care system in the world, but we don't have the healthiest people. We can be, and we should be. It is up to each and every one of us to take health seriously and get on the right path. How you do it is up to you.

Take care of your body. You only have one.

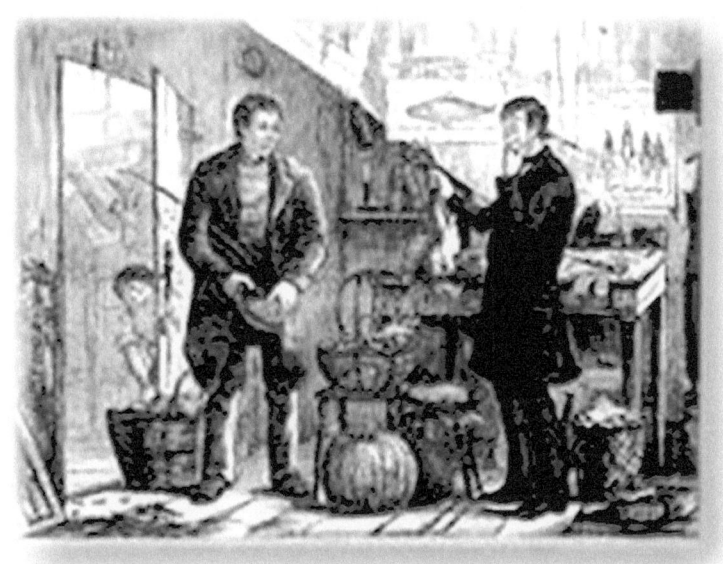

Chapter 10

Bartering Power

Bartering is in your genes. Our ancestors used bartering as an economic means long before money was invented.

The beginnings of commerce in America involved the water powered grain mills. People would bring their grain for grinding into flour. They typically would barter part of their grain for the grinding. The miller would always have surplus grain to sell or barter to someone else. The miller was "top dog" in the community, because he not only had a skill, but also the tools for applying that skill.

Of course that skill was very much in demand. Grain had to be ground for flour and animal feed.

That is what you should be looking for as you build your barter profile. Suffice it to say that, should a major emergency occur in our country, one that lasts for months, anything you have of value to someone else will increase your barter value. These are things necessary for the basic necessities of life and items or services that will increase comfort after the basic necessities are covered. You want to consider things or skills that will be in great demand.

Food will of course be valuable. Seeds might be more valuable. You can buy heirloom seeds *now* for a just a few dollars, $50 would be a good start. They don't take up much space and will be very valuable to barter later. Most seeds available today are hybrid, and hybrid seeds do not produce good seeds for the future. Only open pollinated or heirloom seeds will produce a seed that when planted next year will give you the same results as the parent plant. Hybrid seeds typically produce plants that were created for looks and shipping qualities rather than taste. I find it a shame that some people go to the trouble to grow their own tomatoes, and then at harvest time find that they have the same bland taste as store bought tomatoes. They just purchased the wrong seeds or plants from the nursery. You can find heirloom seeds on the internet. Check and compare because the prices vary greatly.

The Seed Savers Exchange is a good place to start and probably the best place to buy your seeds. You can buy them in small packets or large quantities. Members get a 10% discount, so be sure to join before you buy your seeds. Bulk rates will give you a tremendous discount. For example, a packet of fifty Brandywine tomato seeds cost $2.50, which is cheaper than you can buy them in most stores. You can purchase 1/2 ounce for $27.50, which would make fifty seeds cost about twenty five cents.

If seeds are going to be your barter product, then you need to be an expert on them. Some seeds like onions only keep for one year and others last for several years. Purchase the book, <u>Seed to Seed</u>, from the Seed Savers Exchange at seedsavers.org. Make sure that the seeds you buy are good for your part of the country. The Seed Savers Exchange will help you with that.

The king of all barter products is alcohol. People will go to all lengths to obtain it, and if you have it you can barter it. I mentioned earlier that the beginning of commerce in America was the miller. The tavern was there in the beginning too. Every community had one and many communities grew around where one was located.

Making distilled whisky is probably the most profitable or

barterable, if that is a word. If not, it should be. Whiskey is not that hard to make if you have the right tools. Just like a miller, you need the skill and the tools. Of course, the way to do it and prepare for the future is to start *now*. It is not legal to make whiskey without a permit, but you can get a permit to make it in most states. Do the research and gather your tools of the trade.

You will be able to store corn for use in the mash. This will be the same corn you use for your corn-bread. Just make sure you have enough. Corn is cheap, only about $8 for fifty pounds. Organic corn is much more expensive, but that is the kind I would choose. You can store corn in a dry basement or outbuilding. Make sure you keep it away from rats and mix in diatomaceous earth to keep the bugs at bay.

Beer is definitely the easiest to make. I started making my own beer as research for this book and was surprised at how easy it is. My local brew supply store in Asheville provided everything I needed. It costs about $50 to $100 for the tools and about $30 for the beer kit. For the $30 you can make five gallons of beer which comes to about three dollars a six pack. Not a bad price for a high quality beer. This is the best way to get started. After some experience you can learn the skill of making all-grain beer which brings down your price considerably. With all grain brewing and recycling your yeast, you can brew five gallons of good high quality beer of your choice for under fifteen dollars.

I keg my beer instead of bottling it. I use small five gallon kegs and a freezer with an external thermostat to to keep it around forty two degrees. This is much easier than bottling, but the equipment costs more. Bottling is time consuming. When you bottle your beer, you have to wait two weeks for the beer to carbonize, and I prefer not to wait that long. In a power outage you can store your kegs in a cellar or basement, which keeps the temperature at around fifty eight degrees.

In a nut-shell, beer making is easy. If you can follow directions and boil water, you can make beer.

Wine and hard cider are excellent choices for bartering. Both are easy to make with the right equipment

I think organic fertilizer is a great barter item. Toilet paper will be in demand. Food staples that are dirt cheap now could be very valuable in an emergency. Salt and pepper, some of the cheapest commodities we have, would fit into this category. Salt can be bought in your grocery store for pennies a pound, yet it could easily be worth dollars a pound in an emergency.

If you are a doctor or dentist, prepare your home for items that may be needed by others in an emergency. If you are a welder, keep extra supplies at home. If you have no specialized skills that will be in demand, start working to acquire some *now*. As mentioned earlier, I am studying electrical and electronic technology at my local community college. I think that this skill will be in great demand, especially in hooking up solar panels to houses for electrical needs. Next semester I will be taking welding and will probably buy some welding equipment. I plan to take machining too.

There are numerous skills that will be needed in an emergency. Music will be important. We will probably go back to community barn dances. If you play an instrument, you will have a great barter skill. *Now* is the time to dust off that old guitar or fiddle or whatever you used to play, and start playing music again. You will find that playing that instrument every day will be much more satisfying than sitting in front of the television. If you don't play an instrument, then start lessons *now*. You will be surprised at how quickly you can become proficient at playing a musical instrument when you set your mind to it. And even if you don't use it for barter, you will have something to do to pass the time. Music is relaxing and an enjoyable hobby. It will also enhance your health.

Be creative, and you can come up with many things to barter. I mentioned earlier about learning to make beeswax candles. The key is to do something *now* that will bring you joy and entertainment while making you a little money and preparing you for an uncertain future.

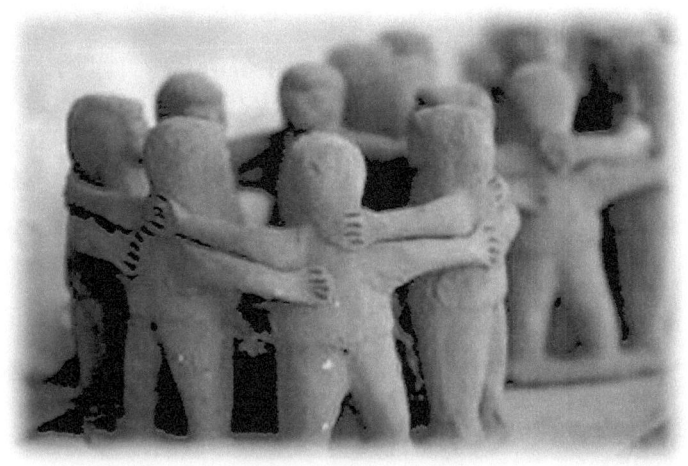

Chapter 11

Community

"No man is an island entire of itself; every man is a piece of the continent, a part of the main".   ...John Donne

"Human beings do not thrive when isolated from others. Donne was a Christian, but this principal is shared by other religions."

...skysmom65

Communities are important. Communities are what helped mankind survive for all of history. No man is an island. This is a profound truth that transcends time. Only in the last 100 years have many of us lost this precious sense of community. Deep down we crave it, and yet we aren't even aware of this gnawing addiction to our souls.

Many of us have it now. Our churches provide a tremendous community atmosphere. But so many people on this earth today have very little sense of community. It is probably a contributing factor to some of our illnesses and addictions.

We will need communities in a disaster more than ever. People will survive in isolation, but people will flourish in a community. The community helps us receive everything we need, from our food to our companionship. We need each other, and if you don't believe that, try going without human contact for three months. You will get very lonely, and your immune system will suffer.

The people of Ikaria Island in Greece are among the longest living and healthiest people in the world. Along with a diet rich with organic greens, whole grains and fresh vegetables, their social community is noted as being a strong contributing factor for their vibrant health.

In Ikaria families live together or close to each other. They have very strong social networks and close friends, no matter what their age. The elderly and young hang out together. The elderly participate in all activities. This community bond has been attributed to good health in many other cultures as well.

A study from Harvard University links friendships with increased brain function. A study from Australia points to an increase in longevity to having friendships in old age. Community and social networks contribute to the health and long lives of Okinawans of Japan and the Hunzas of Pakistan.

Those of you who can afford it should look at having a place where you can go to escape the highly populated areas. A cabin in the mountains surrounded by friends and family would be ideal. Choose the right land and location. Make sure that the property is isolated enough to insure privacy.

How about 10 or more families or groups of people joining together to create a wonderful little mini village? One where white collar workers would work together with blue collar workers to create an ideal community, knowing that all are best served by involving people and interacting with people from different walks of life. People with different skills who "bring something to the table", working and sharing common goals make the best communities. I can imagine a community with a doctor, a dentist, a welder, a brewer, a master gardener, a beautician, and electrician, a plumber, a massage therapist, teachers, mechanics, etc and so on and on. The more the merrier, but small is good, too.

This is not a commune. I do not advocate community property, but in a disaster there is no doubt that a commune will work better than no community at all. I prefer to think that a common sharing community with individual barteristic principles would be best. Barterism would replace capitalism. But unlike capitalism, there is no greed in barterism. In a barteristic community, greed is not only absent, it is counter-productive therefore making it obsolete. It simply cannot exist.

Start planning with your friends and family. You never know where this may lead. You might think you cannot afford it, but with a little creativity and some planning you might be surprised.

There are plenty of areas in the rural countryside that are inexpensive. Three or more families could sell their urban or suburban homes and buy 100 acres, build 900 sq. ft. homes and start a community. Or maybe share one house for a while, and then build from there. It is better to live in a 400 sq. ft. house and be self-sufficient and happy, surrounded by friends, than to live in a mansion with fear and loneliness.

It is time to get your friends and family involved. Should a disaster come, you want all your friends and family to be prepared. Here is a statement that I have to repeat.

You must make every attempt to help your family and friends prepare *now*.

You will not have enough to go around, and you might have to make some unpleasant and tough choices if a disaster should come. The easiest way to get them involved is to show them what you are doing. This is a more effective way of convincing others than preaching to them. Make them a little envious. Give them a glimpse of what you are doing and a small taste of your new confidence. Show them that you are having fun while getting prepared. Peak their interest by teasing them with a few tidbits of information about your preparation. If you keep it elusive and a little bit secretive, you will arouse their attention more.

Invite them to experience some of your new lifestyle changes. Have a fresh bread party. Include them in grinding grain and making bread. Have some ready to pop into the oven. Help them enjoy and experience this wonderful smelling and tasting of fresh whole-wheat bread. Add a few healthy spreads, like garlic hummus or basil spread with sun dried tomatoes. Maybe introduce them to some of your own brewed beer or hard cider. Show them how you can cook pinto beans in your pressure cooker in under ten minutes.

151

You will be pleased at how impressed they are with your new healthy lifestyle.

This will be a good time to introduce them into doing the same. There is nothing more powerful than peer pressure. Not that you will be pressuring them, but just the evidence of what you are doing will be enough.

The more friends and family you have involved, the easier it will be on you. You may be the one to start the trend toward a healthier more sustainable lifestyle. There is no better way to prepare for the future than getting your significant others involved. You will be helping them start a healthier lifestyle while reinforcing your own decisions. You will be helping them prepare for the future and encouraging them to make the best decisions of their lives for a healthier and happier today.

In an emergency you will be satisfied that people you love and care for are prepared. Hopefully they will introduce others to this lifestyle. This trend could go viral, and I hope it will. If everyone made the commitment to start *now* and bring their friends and family on board, we all would benefit.

This great country, which has been sliding a bit down the road to mediocrity, will again lead the world in health and happiness. We will be more confident. Nothing makes you feel more confident than being in control of every aspect of your life.

What more could you ask for?   Working together with your friends and family toward common goals, bonding as you attain a level of self-sufficiency, is an achievement of health and joy. Getting your hands dirty and making things happen, bonding with Mother Earth, feeling the health benefits of your efforts, watching your loved ones flourish.....these and more can be yours as you take this new lifestyle one step at a time.

The benefits are endlessly satisfying. Instead of mindless television mediocrity, why not go down to the basement and brew some beer? Why not go back to the local community college and learn a skill? Why not meet with friends and form a prepare club? Why not have fun doing it?

As I sit here writing this, thousands of protestors are "occupying Wall Street" in cities and towns all across the United States. They are protesting the great disparity of income in the United States, the loss of the middle class and the greed that has brought our magnificent country to its knees. They are protesting the powerless feeling that a few billionaires are in control of our lives. They are protesting a feeling of helplessness, that it is no longer within our power to do anything about it.

What better way to protest than to become healthy and sustainable? What better way to show the 1% mega-zillionaires and the mega-businesses that greedily feed us poisons and toxins on a daily basis that we don't need them.

Let us redefine our message from "We won't take it anymore"; to "We don't need you anymore." Nothing could grab their attention better. Nothing could affect our true economy and our true self-respect as a nation as profoundly as becoming more self-sustainable, more reliable on ourselves, and having more self-confidence in our ability to survive. When we prepare and become more sustainable, we gain a confidence that many of us have never experienced. We know we can survive regardless of what comes our way.

What would Wall Street do if we decided not to have Christmas this year in the conventional commercial way? What if we decided to spiritually celebrate Christmas this year in the most moving way that each citizen chooses, regardless of religion? What if we decided as a nation of good-minded citizens that it would be in our best interest to make our own Christmas gifts or buy them locally without credit cards and not at large department stores?

I am not advocating protest. I am advocating change from the status quo. I am suggesting a shift of power from the powerless to becoming the powerful. When people know that they can provide for their needs, and know their neighbors can provide for their needs, and know that together they can help each other, power is achieved.

Ok, I have rambled again and gotten off track a little. My point is start *now* and do what you can. Have a sincere and heartfelt meeting with your family and decide to spend less on useless material things and use the extra money to prepare. The ones who take heed and prepare will benefit *now*.

And *now* is all there is.

There is no better time.

There is no other time.

There is a New Earth and it is upon us. It may take a disaster to move some people to this new way of living and thinking. Many will embrace it and make the change naturally, because this New Earth is what our souls are craving.

Selfishness and greed have no place in this New Earth. Bullying and pride are being replaced by sharing and cooperation.

Corporations are now beginning to understand that people are what make them great... their own employees and the people they serve. The corporations that resist may cease to exist.

In the New Earth people are accepted for who they are, regardless of race, religion or ideals. Wars are unnecessary. Peace will prevail. We are finally realizing that we are all connected.

In this New Earth,

The Golden Rule rules.

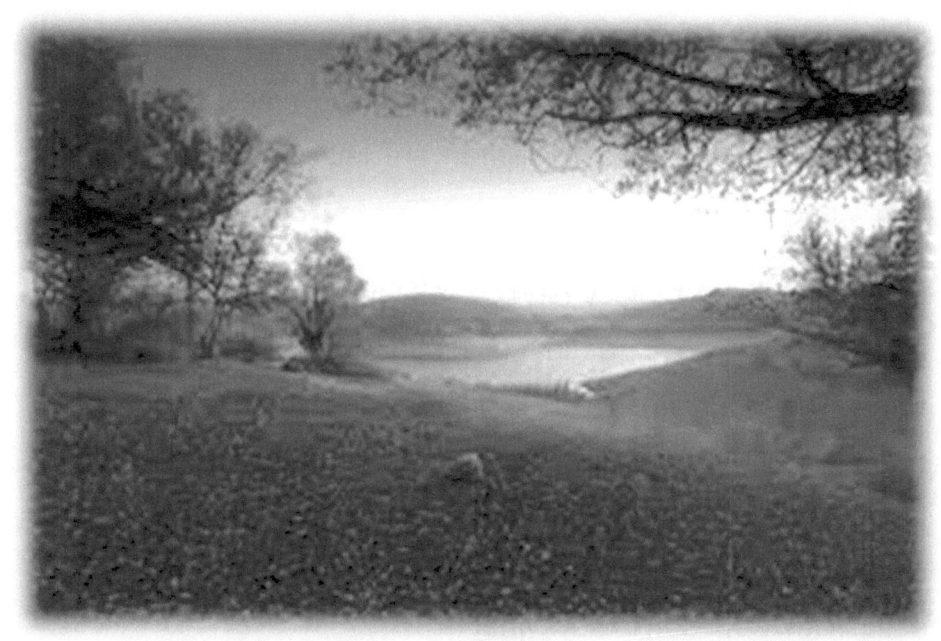

Conclusion

Chapter 12

A s I end this book, I want to tell you a story about an enchanted land.

Here is a land where there is no cancer, where men and women live a vigorous life at 100 or 120 years of age. This is a land where optometrists find that everyone has 20-20 vision. Cardiologists cannot find a trace of coronary heart disease.. This is a land where men father children at ninety years old.

The inhabitants are the happiest people in the world. They get together each evening and play games. Even the 90-year-olds participate. Children are taught values of love, family and community.

Sound like a fantasy land? In fact it is very real. It is a place called Hunza, a tiny community in Pakistan, in the Himalayan Mountains. This is a land where there is no crime, no money, no generation gaps and no stores. These people have enjoyed super health for 2,000 years. If that is not enough to perk up our attention and motivate us to take a look at this lifestyle, I don't know what is.

Maybe you think this is all a well traveled rumor, that there really is no land or people like this. Well, think again. In the 1960s an optometrist, Dr. Allen E. Banik, made the journey to see for himself if these people were for real. He discovered that all of this was true.

Two cardiologists, Dr. Paul White and Dr. Edward Toomey, also made a journey to find out for themselves. They took along a battery-operated electrocardiograph. They reported their findings in the American Heart Journal in December of 1964. After testing 25 men who appeared to be between 90 and 110 years old by good evidence, they found no high blood pressure, no elevated levels of cholesterol and no signs of coronary disease.

The ninety-year-old men work every day, play a game very similar to volleyball with men fifty years younger, and a type of polo game that is physically difficult, similar to rugby.

To study what causes this amazing feat of health, we need to look at not only what they eat, but what they don't eat.

They don't eat food processed with chemicals. They don't eat food that was grown by someone thousands of miles away. They don't eat food with preservatives or plastic packaging. They don't eat lots of meat. They don't eat meat from factory farms laden with antibiotics just to keep the animal alive long enough for slaughter. The meat they eat is what we consider organic free range. They don't have a name for organic because it is the only way they raise their food.

They eat only fresh and naturally preserved food. Their food processing is drying fresh fruits in the sun and making butter and cheese from goat's milk. They use no chemicals or artificial fertilizer. In fact it is against Hunza law to use pesticides.

Once when told to spray their orchards by Pakistani officials because of an impending insect invasion, they refused. Instead they treated their trees with an organic mixture of ashes and water, which protected their crops without using poison.

One of their favorite foods is apricots. They eat them fresh in season and dry them for the future. They even make an ice cream out of dried apricots and snow, with no sugar since the dried apricots are sweet enough without it. Then they eat the seeds. The women hand grind these then press them to make oil. They use the oil for cooking, for their lamps and even for a skin cream.

They eat lots of fruits and vegetables, mostly raw because fuel is rare and precious. They sprout their seeds, gaining important nutrients. These sprouts contain high levels of nitrilosides, also known as vitamin B17. Some believe that nitrilosides may be to cancer what vitamin C is to scurvy.

They eat fresh bread, saving the grain and grinding it at the time of making the bread. Their grains consist of millet, buckwheat, wheat and barley.

The bottom line is that they are in touch with their food. They are in touch with their community.

They are in touch with life, and it shows.

We can follow their example and get in touch with our food, our communities and our lives. As we prepare for an uncertain future, we can light our path with healthy alternatives, and make those the rule rather than the exception.

Good luck on your journey. I hope you bring many others
along with you.

Here is a list of books and references for your library.

Healthy Bread in Five Minutes a Day

Artisan Bread in Five Minutes a Day

by Jeff Hertzberg, M.D., and Zoe Francois

Mother Earth News   motherearthnews.com

One Second After by William R. Forstchen

Gardening When It Counts by Steve Solomon

Square Foot Gardening by Mel Bartholomew

Pressure Cooking ,The Easy Way by Maureen B. Keane and Daniella

Chace

Food Drying With an Attitude by Mary T. Bell

BackPack Gourmet by Linda Frederick Yaffe

New Earth Shelters newearthshelters.com

SumHouse sumhouse.org

Mountain Green Builders mtngreenbuilders.com

The Great Disruption: Why the Climate Crisis Will Bring on the End of Shopping and the Birth of New World   Paul Gilding

A New Earth: Awakening to Your Life's Purpose   Eckhart Tolle

For more information please check out our website at

www.howtopreparenow.com

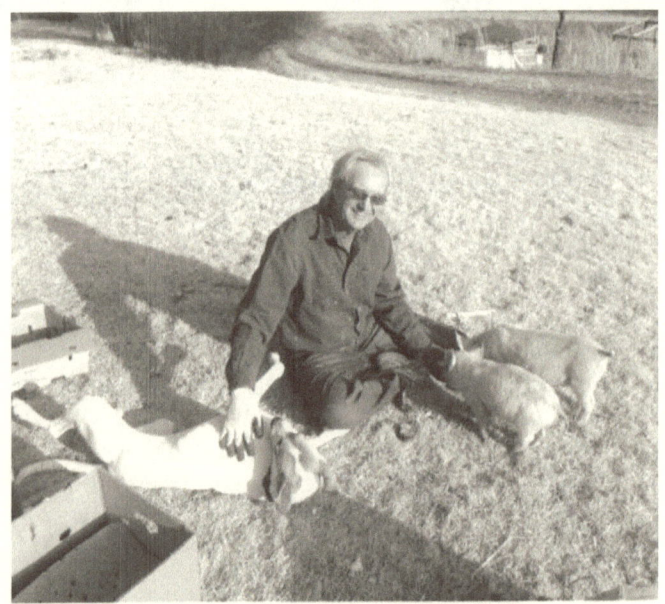

ABOUT THE AUTHOR

Larry Deal lives in Old Fort, North Carolina. He has a degree in psychology from Western Carolina University. Larry is a general contractor and specializes in strong, sustainable, energy efficient structures.

You can contact Larry at www.howtopreparenow.com

www.ingramcontent.com/pod-product-compliance
Lightning Source LLC
Chambersburg PA
CBHW020427290526
45785CB00002B/727